Sports Medicine

For

Moms

Sports Medicine for Moms: How to feel confident deciding when to get immediate medical care, when to wait, and what care to give at home by Deniece Oates, MS, ATC

Published by Deniece Oates
Home Sports Medicine
www.homesportsmed.com

Cover design and formatting by Philemon Eniola
Edited by Rachel Garber

ISBN: 978-1-7376786-0-1
ISBN: 978-1-7376786-1-8

Disclaimer

The information provided in this book is designed to provide helpful information on the subjects discussed. This book is not meant to be used, nor should it be used, to diagnose or treat any medical condition. For diagnosis or treatment of any medical problem, consult your own physician, who can address the problem using the facts and circumstances of your individual situation. The publisher and author are not responsible for any injury needs that may require medical supervision and are not liable for any damages or negative consequences from any treatment, action, application or preparation, to any person reading or following the information in this book. References are provided for informational purposes only and do not constitute endorsement of any websites or other sources. Readers should be aware that the websites listed in this book may change.

A Note about Supplies

In this book, you will find many items mentioned that are particularly useful in the care of sports injuries. These supplies are best kept on hand, so you don't have to stress about finding them when you need them!

There is no "First Aid Kit" that gathers all of these supplies in one - so I'm working on that! In the meantime, I have created a list of these recommended supplies with links to where you can buy them.

Check out Home Sports Medicine's **On the Go Sports Injury Care Kit Supply Recommendations List** at: www.homesportsmed.com

TABLE OF CONTENTS

Disclaimer i

Introduction v

What Happens When an Injury Occurs? 1

What Counts as an Emergency 4

What to do if it's Not an Emergency 9

What to Use to Ice 18

What to Use to Heat up 21

Fractures 24

Dislocations 31

Concussions 36

Common Shoulder Injuries 63

Low Back, Hamstring, IT Band, Groin and Hip Flexor Muscle Injuries 69

Deep Bruises 79

Common Knee Injuries 82

Shin Splints 91

Common Ankle Injuries 94

Blisters 98

Bruises Toenails 100

Dehydrations and Heat Illness 102

Cuts, Lacerations and Abrasions 110

Conclusion 116

INTRODUCTION

When I went into Sports Medicine, I knew there would always be a need for it. Injuries are a given in sports and activities, and people of all ages love to play. I have family, friends and neighbors asking me on a regular basis for help and advice with various problems. Taking care of injuries properly makes returning to normal daily function and then to playing sports again so much easier. Mishandling them can complicate your life forever after.

As a parent, making decisions about what care to seek out and provide when your child is injured can be complicated. It's hard to tell, for example, if a child's reaction to an injury is a useful measure of how serious the problem is. It's hard to know how to get the best care for the money you have to pay, and even how to prioritize cost relative to long-term consequences. It's difficult to make decisions for your child, when you don't really know what, exactly, they are experiencing, what's really wrong, and what your treatment options are. It's particularly overwhelming, in the moments right after an injury, when you have to decide what to do. You certainly don't want to make a bad choice, and cause further problems or damage.

This book comes from over 25 years of experience taking care of sports injuries, and is meant to help parents feel more confident about knowing when an injury requires urgent medical care, when professional evaluation can wait for a less urgent, less expensive setting, and when you can handle things well enough at home. When you know what specific signs to look for, and what specific steps to take, decisions can be much easier and much less stressful to make. Knowing what care to give will ease pain, promote a return to full function, limit the damage from an injury, and optimize your child's longer term prognosis. Some essential knowledge will lessen stress and worry for you and for your child. You are the one who is with your child the most — care you provide can be the best and most helpful!

Injuries are difficult — there's no getting around that fact. But I have learned over many years and with hundreds of young athletes, that the choices you make in the first minutes, hours, and days after an injury can either make things much worse or make the recovery process as smooth and quick as possible. The care you give immediately after an injury makes all the difference in the outcome.

WHAT HAPPENS WHEN AN INJURY OCCURS?

This depends on the injury and can be a very complicated process, but I offer here the basic and almost universal ways the body responds to injury. These are essential to understand when your goal is to minimize damage from an injury and create the best possible conditions for healing and recovery.

Below are four general phases of the injury and healing process:

1 - Hemostasis and Inflammation

Hemostasis is the process the body goes through to contain and stop bleeding that happens when an injury occurs, both inside and on the surface of the body. When any body tissue is stressed and damaged, individual cells die either from direct damage, or because the flow of blood and oxygen that feeds them is interrupted. When blood vessels tear open, blood and other damaged tissue cells leak into the surrounding area. Chemicals from the damaged tissue initiate the process of blood clotting to stop the leakage. Active bleeding must be stopped before any clean up or healing can begin. The clotting process can happen quickly or go on for several hours or even days, depending on how much damage there is, and if any intervention is applied.

At the same time the body is working to control the bleeding caused by an injury, inflammation also occurs. The process of Inflammation is characterized by chemicals released by the damaged tissue causing pain and muscle spasm. This reaction is your body's effort to minimize further injury. Swelling, another characteristic of inflammation, builds as long as fluid leakage continues. This causes pain due to pressure build-up, and redness and heat due to the amount of blood in the area. At the end of this stage, cells are attracted to the area that do the work of cleaning out any dead cells and any foreign matter that has accumulated. Inflammation lasts from a few hours to several days, depending on the amount of initial damage, and how the injury is treated in this crucial time.

To give an example of what you see when this process is happening, I'll use an ankle sprain, the most common injury in sports. An ankle sprain occurs when the foot is forced into a position that is beyond its normal available motion. When this happens, ligaments stretch and tear. Ligaments are the structures that attach the bones to each other. The tears can be small or large. When ligaments tear, blood vessels break, causing blood and ligament tissue cells to flow into the surrounding area. Chemicals released by the torn tissue cause the sensation of pain, and cause the surrounding muscles to tighten up. This helps reduce the risk of further injury by limiting mobility. The ankle and surrounding area of the foot and lower leg swell, or get bigger, as blood and cells continue to flow from the torn tissue. Swelling causes more pain from the buildup of pressure and also limits the motion available at the foot and ankle. The area flushes red and gets warm, because of the increased presence of blood. Discoloration can appear after a day or two. How much discoloration depends on the amount of the damage.

2 - Rebuilding and repair

Chemicals released in the area of injury attract other cells to the site whose purpose is to rebuild and repair. While bone cells are repaired with the same cells as the original ones, all other damaged tissue (skin, ligament, tendon, muscle) is filled in by scar tissue. Scar tissue is not as strong or as flexible as the original tissue, and the body tends to overdo the deployment of scar tissue, just to make sure the area gets covered. Treatment and rehabilitation are especially useful at this time, to help the body lay down scar tissue in an ideal way, which will allow for normal movement. Without proper treatment and rehabilitation, an injury can create problems with limited motion and inefficient patterns of muscle contraction that persist for a long time. Lack of appropriate treatment and rehab increases the likelihood of further injury or reinjury in the future. The rebuilding phase can last from a few days to several weeks. The injured area is especially vulnerable to reinjury during this time.

During this period, the swelling associated with a sprained ankle will gradually go down, though it may never be the same size as the uninjured ankle again. Discoloration will go from blue/purple to shades of green, then fade away. As scar tissue is laid down, pain will dissipate with normal activities and motion will improve.

3 - Remodeling

This phase lasts several weeks to months, and can even take years. The scar tissue is strengthened and modified. Scar tissue, however, will never be as strong or flexible as the original tissue, as it is less organized at a cellular level. It is very important to continue to protect the body part through this phase with taping, sleeves, braces, etc. It is also very important during this period to strengthen the surrounding muscles and retrain efficient patterns of muscle firing. This retraining happens through a rehabilitation program. If it's done correctly, it will produce efficient motion, allowing the body to return to normal function.

It's common for people to shortchange the remodeling phase. Not much is noticeable from the outside during this process, and when people get to the point that they can return to regular daily activities, they assume the injury is healed. Returning to full athletic function, however, requires a higher level of strength and ideal efficiency in patterns of muscle firing. Performing at peak levels of speed, power, and agility will not happen without further treatment and rehabilitation during this phase, and the injured body part will be vulnerable to reinjury due to lack of ideal function.
https://www.ncbi.nlm.nih.gov/books/NBK3938/

WHAT COUNTS AS AN EMERGENCY?

An emergency means you need to get professional medical care as soon as possible - but there are some things to take into consideration about where to go and how much to spend getting there. How do you know what absolutely requires an ER visit? How do you know if you need to get there by ambulance or if you can safely drive your child there yourself? In the panic of the moment, parents tend to make the most conservative choice. They don't want to harm their child just to save the cost of an ambulance ride. Understanding the risk involved and knowing what your options are will let you make the best choice, for your child and for your finances. Here are some guidelines to help you decide quickly what situations require an ER visit and whether you need an ambulance to get there.

EMERGENCIES THAT REQUIRE AN AMBULANCE

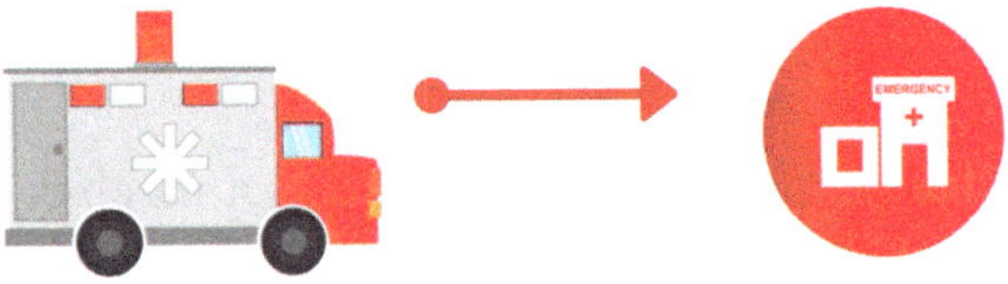

First off, the big ones:

Not breathing

Requires rescue breathing ASAP

The heart is not beating

Requires CPR ASAP

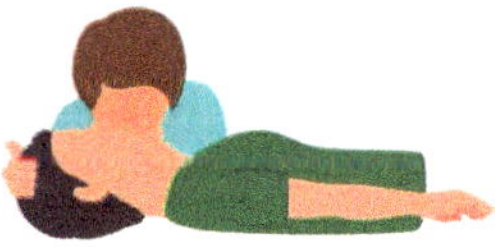
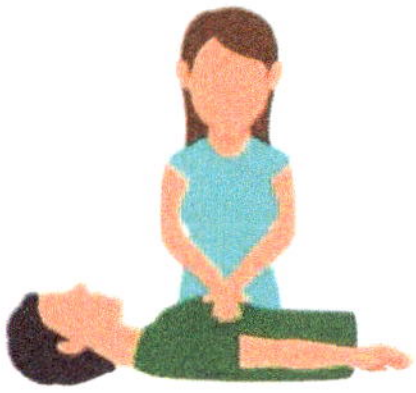
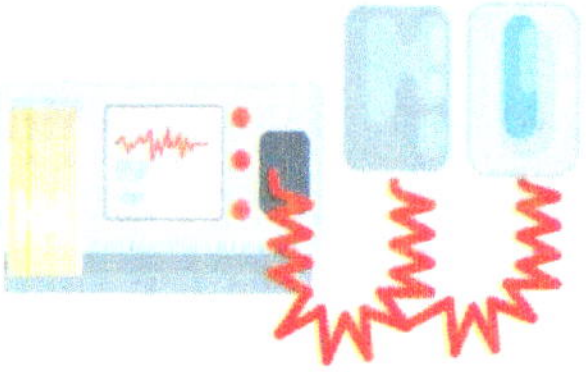

An ambulance brings with it paramedics or EMT's that are certified to do both of those things - but more importantly, they will have an **AED** (Automated External Defibrillator), a machine that has a much higher rate of successful resuscitation than CPR/rescue breathing alone (more than double).

The next biggest ones:

Obvious spinal cord damage

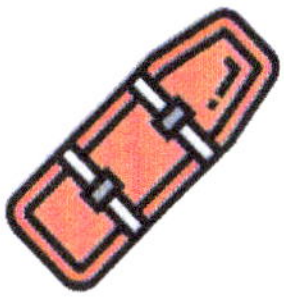

You should assume spinal cord damage if the athlete tells you they can't move or feel a body part, that feeling comes and goes, or there is a tingling or burning sensation.

Unconsciousness that lasts longer than 1 minute

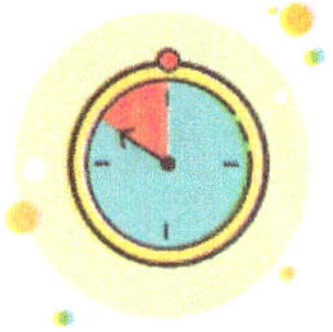

This involves a brain injury and you must also assume there is a spinal cord injury, as you cannot prove otherwise.

Blood and/or clear liquid coming out of the mouth, ears, eyes or nose

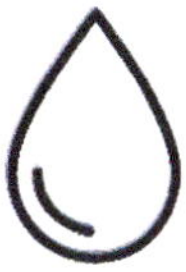

Blood and/or clear liquid coming out of the ears, nose, or mouth indicate a serious head injury. This is different from a simple bloody nose.

Major concussion symptoms, or symptoms that quickly get worse

Major concussion symptoms include

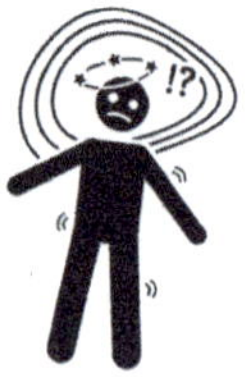

- Seizures or convulsions
- Deteriorating state of consciousness
- Vomiting
- Major and increasing headache

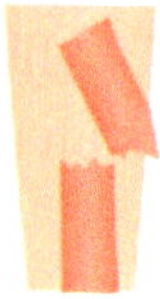

Compound fracture (broken bone sticking out through the skin). Compound fractures are often associated with extensive bleeding - a lot of it and fast. This bleeding is usually difficult to stop.

The following injuries may not look as serious, so the question of how to handle them is less obvious, but they too require a trip to the ER and in an ambulance:

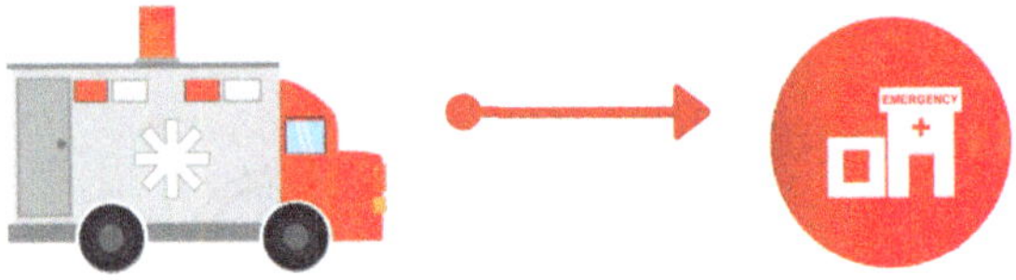

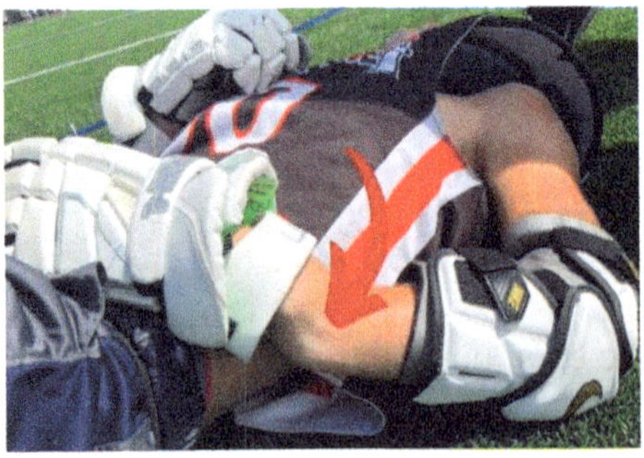

Fractures where there is obvious deformity:

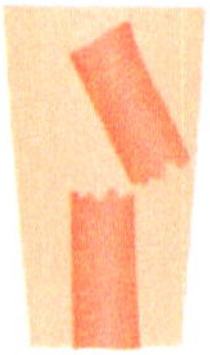

These don't break through the skin, and won't usually involve external bleeding, but if there are odd angles, or something doesn't look right, don't mess with it. Moving it around can cause further damage, or damage to other structures.

Dislocations that stay out of place - accompanied by interruption of blood flow or nerve conduction

Dislocations that stay out of place will look deformed. Interruption of blood flow can be seen by changes in skin coloring below the affected body part. If you pinch a finger or toe, and it stays white, instead of filling in to a natural color again, you should assume interrupted blood flow. A nerve conduction problem would be manifested by abnormal sensation, such as pins and needles, or numbness.

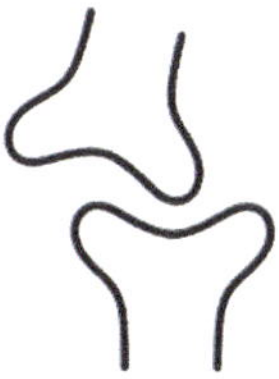

Shock

All serious injuries, and even some moderate injuries involve shock to some degree. It is the effect of insufficient blood flow in the core body area due to blood pooling in the extremities. Symptoms include rapid, shallow breathing, rapid, weak pulse and cold, clammy skin. It is best to anticipate this and take steps to aid blood circulation by propping the legs up, if the situation allows it, and keeping the athlete warm with jackets or a blanket.

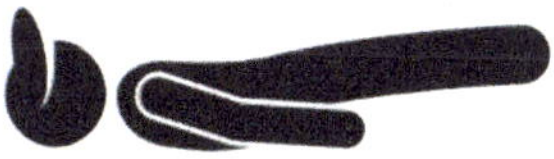

The following injuries require immediate medical care. Call a sports medicine physician's office first, just to see if you can get in quickly. If not, you can drive the athlete to the Urgent Care or ER.

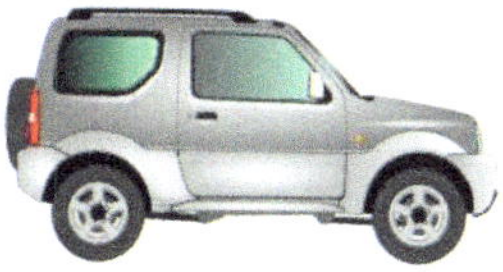

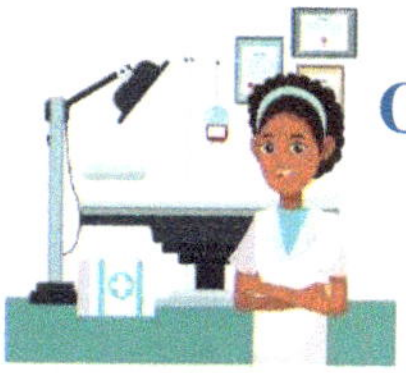

OR

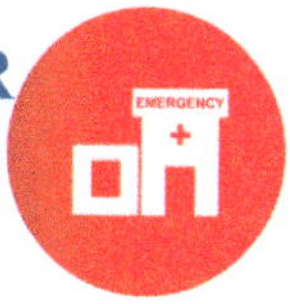

Dislocations that stay out of place, but do not have a problem with blood flow or nerve conduction

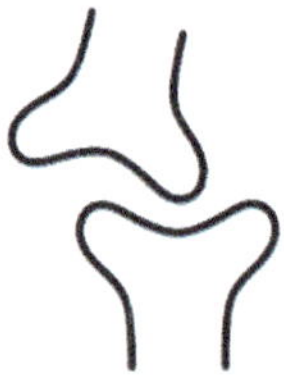

There is no change of skin coloring in the body part, and no abnormal sensation, but a lot of pain! See the section on dislocations (p. 31) for what to do for immediate care.

Concussion symptoms that progressively get worse or stay the same, within several hours of injury

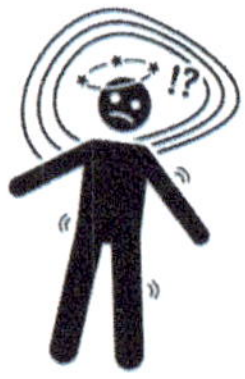

Most concussion signs and symptoms start to clear away within an hour or so of injury, though it is common to have a few that come and go for many days. If, however, any concussion symptoms get worse or there are several symptoms that stay the same, go get checked out right away. See the section on concussions (p. 35) for information on what symptoms to watch for and a way to keep track of them.

Stitches

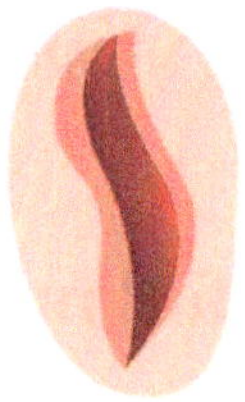

Try the doctor's office first, but if it's after hours or on the weekend, head to the Urgent Care or ER. See the section on Cuts, Abrasions and Lacerations (p. 92) for more details on how to decide what needs stitches, and for initial care instructions.

WHAT TO DO IF IT'S NOT AN EMERGENCY

If an injury doesn't fit in the above listing of what needs immediate professional medical care, it still needs immediate care, but YOU can provide it - actually better than an ER or Urgent Care! A doctor visit might still be needed, but it can wait a few days until you can get an appointment. In some cases, a visit to the doctor may not even be necessary if you provide good early care in the first few days after the injury. You'll be able to make that determination by following the guidelines outlined below and watching carefully for the outcome.

RICE - the go to care for the first 24-72 hours

You may already be familiar with the acronym RICE:

R = Rest
I = Ice
C = Compression
E = Elevation

All of these interventions are aimed at reducing the possibility of further injury and influencing the extent to which the inflammatory process, the body's natural response to injury, is allowed to go on. There is a logic in not cutting off the natural inflammatory process too much - it is an important part of the healing process. The interventions described below simply moderate the response. This helps with pain and enables a quicker return to function. I can say from experience, that without any intervention, the body's natural inflammatory response will cause the healing process to take much longer than it will if intervention occurs. I can best explain how this works using the analogy of a series of hoses.

The Hose Analogy

Think of your blood vessels as a series of hoses delivering water to several different stations in an enclosed space. Imagine that a particular section of hose gets damaged and starts leaking water into the surrounding area. The first thing you have to do is stop whatever is causing the damage to the hose. Resting an injured body part stops whatever caused the damage to begin with and limits further damage.

The next step is to repair the damaged hose. You can't turn off the water all together, as it is imperative that each station has a consistent supply. You therefore have to patch the hose while water is still flowing through it.

You can imagine that it will be difficult to apply a patch and get it to stick with water flowing swiftly through it and squirting everywhere. Patching will be a lot easier if you can at least slow the flow. You've got several options to do this.

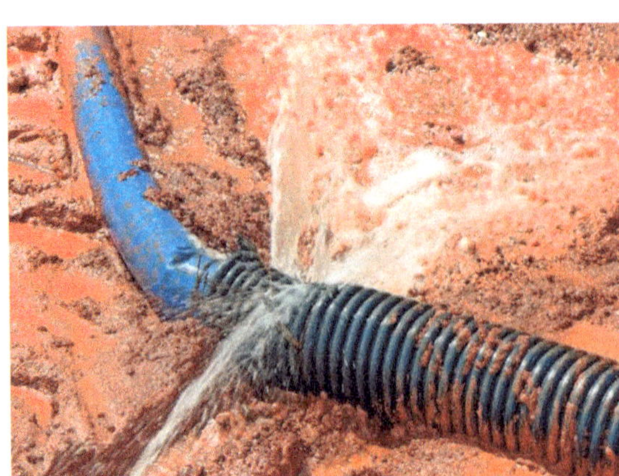

One option is to lower the temperature in the damaged area. The viscosity of water will increase as its temperature decreases, increasing the friction between the water and the wall of the hose. This will slow the rate of flow. This is the effect of ice on a damaged body area. Naturally, when movement through one area is slowed, a large amount of water will automatically flow into other avenues where it is allowed to move more quickly.

Another way to slow the flow is constrict or apply mild pressure to the area immediately around the damaged hose. This makes for a smaller space through which the water can pass. A greater percentage of water will automatically be routed through different sections that remain more open, and less will pass through the constricted area. Applying compression to a damaged body part moderates the blood flow through the damaged area.

The last option for limiting flow is to make gravity work for you. Elevation of the hose causes the water to have to flow upward, which makes it harder and therefore slower. Elevation of a damaged body part means that the blood will have to push uphill to get to the damaged area and can be a useful way to moderate the amount of blood moving through it.

With any injury to body tissue, blood vessels are torn. Torn vessels allow blood and damaged cells to leak out into the surrounding tissue where they don't belong. This is what causes swelling. Stopping the bleeding is the body's number one priority, therefore the process of clotting begins immediately. How long it lasts depends on the amount of damage and how diligently interventions are applied. The purpose of rest, ice, compression and elevation is to slow down blood flow through the injured area, which will allow the body to more quickly clot off the damaged blood vessels. It will not stop the flow entirely, and some leaking will go on, which will activate the body's normal inflammatory response. The healing process cannot begin, however, until the bleeding has stopped.

Back to the analogy with the damaged hose - how much water leaks out if interventions are applied, and the patching process takes 6 hours, as opposed to how much water will have leaked out if no interventions are applied and the patching process takes 24 hours? The damage to the hose isn't any greater in the 24 hour scenario than the 6 hour scenario, but the amount of water that leaked out and now has to be cleaned up and pumped out is vastly greater.

Blood and damaged cells outside of the circulatory system have to be cycled out of the body through the garbage - the lymph system, which is an amazing process, but it takes time. Limiting the amount of blood that leaks out of damaged blood vessels and into the surrounding tissue simply means that there will be less garbage to take out. It does not mean that chemicals and processes triggered by the presence of blood outside the blood vessels will not come at all or not enough of them will come to produce full healing of damaged tissues.

Remember our damaged hose is in a contained area, which means that pressure builds up as more and more water leaks out. This not only hampers the patching process, it makes cleaning up more difficult, which in turn causes it to take more time.

The pressure exerted by blood leaking out of damaged vessels and building up in the surrounding tissues is an important negative factor in injury because it causes a lot of pain. For the purposes of this discussion, however, it is important because it hampers the clean up process in that it squeezes off small lymph collector vessels, making them inefficient at carrying out their job of cycling the unwanted fluid out.

How to apply the interventions of RICE:

Rest:

The purpose of rest is to protect the injured body part from further damage due to ongoing use or delayed care. While pain associated with a serious injury necessitates rest, an injury that is not as serious is often ignored, in order to get through the game, or get through work or school. Rest doesn't just mean sitting on the couch, watching TV, and

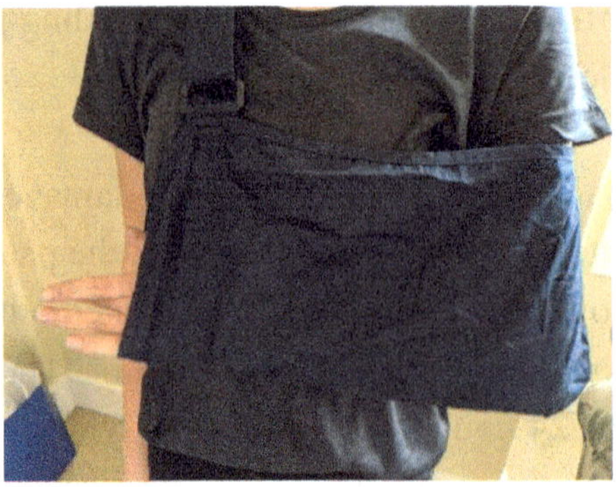

expecting someone to keep the snacks coming. It also includes the use of crutches or a brace or sling. Depending on the injury, a compromise can be made about when these aids need to be used and for how long.

Rest always includes getting the full amount of recommended sleep and also some additional time. Sleep time is when most healing occurs.

Ice:

For the first 24-72 hours:

Ice for 20 minutes on and about 1.5 hours off, as often as you can (don't wake up at night to put ice on)
DO NOT sit in a hot tub or take a warm bath with the body part immersed in water during this time frame (A quick warm shower is OK). Heat has the opposite effect as ice, so blood flow will increase into the area.

Compression:

Ace bandage:

Wrap an ace bandage starting at the point of the body part furthest from the heart, and wrap towards the heart. Remember the compression will limit blood flow into the area, so any body part below the ace bandage will have blood that pools in it, causing it to swell. That is why the ankle wrap starts at the toes, the knee wrap starts at the ankle, and an arm wrap starts

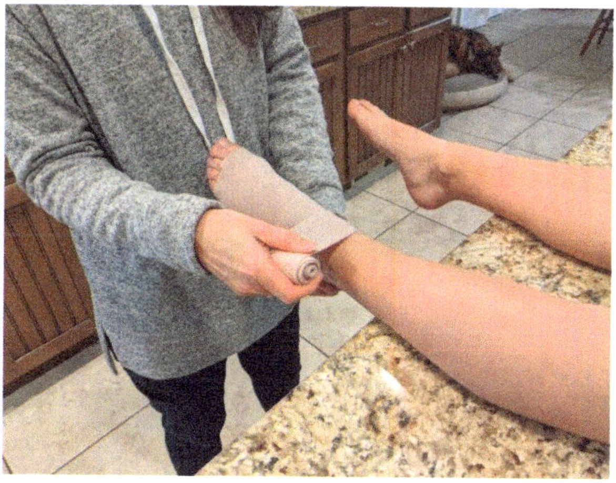

down at the wrist. The wrap should be tight until it passes the injured area, then whatever of the bandage is left can be loose. You can check whether the bandage is too tight by pinching the tip of a toe or finger below the wrap. **The place where you pinch should get white when pinched, but fill in to normal color again quickly.** If the pinched area doesn't return to normal color, the bandage is too tight.

Also, be aware that injuries tend to throb at night. This leads many people to take off the bandage and then wake up with a lot of swelling! The bandage can be loosened in the case of throbbing, but don't take it completely off.

To watch a video showing how to apply an ace bandage click one of the following links:

Knee injury: https://youtu.be/oMsAURiOjj4

Ankle injury: https://youtu.be/UmcSrN99_Qw

Hand, wrist, forearm injury:
https://youtu.be/0wvPUHSk0hE

Sleeve:

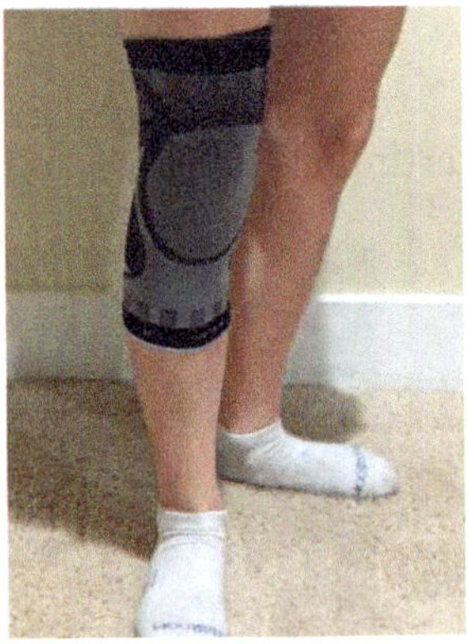

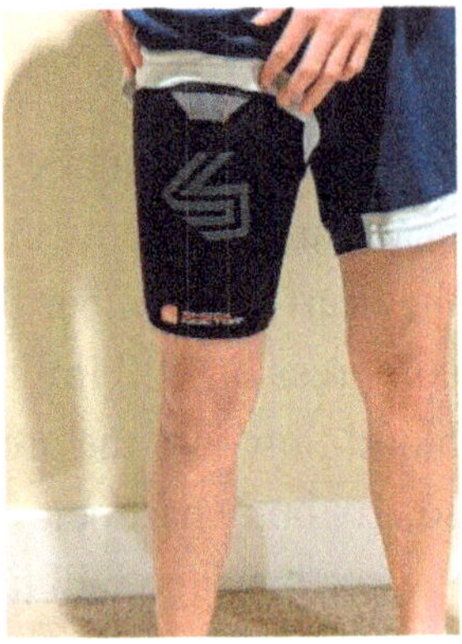

A sleeve made out of neoprene or compression knit material can also provide compression. Though they may cause some swelling in the body parts below them, one advantage they have over ace bandages is being a little more comfortable to wear. This can help an injured athlete be more willing to wear it. Sleeves are best for thighs, knees or elbows.

Elevation:

Sit or lie with the body part above the heart. If that is not possible, at least keep the body part off the ground and lifted as much as possible. This is the case for arms too, so find a way to prop the arm up that is comfortable.

Pain relief:

Acetaminophen is your best over-the-counter option in this initial stage of the injury. The reason is that it is a pain reliever, but not an anti-inflammatory, such as ibuprofen. One of the properties of anti-inflammatories is that they thin the blood. While an injury is in the stage of active bleeding and the body is working on clotting off damaged blood vessels, thinning the blood causes more bleeding, counter to the purpose.

The mental game:

The perspective and attitude of the athlete plays a significant role in recovery from injury and a confident return to play. How you approach the athlete and the injury during this time is crucial to positively moving forward. There is a balance to be found in recognizing the severity of a problem and acting accordingly, but not over dramatising in one direction or playing it down in the other. It is so so hard to watch your child struggle with physical and emotional pain, but you will make it harder by having an overly dramatic reaction to what the injury looks like or the lack of function the child has. Hopefully, keeping in mind that your reaction will influence the response of the child will help you keep the dramatics in check! Shrugging an injury off or encouraging the child to discount what they are feeling will also lead to a dysfunctional response and a less-than-ideal healing process. Strive to be calm, speak positively but realistically, and encourage compliance. This is a game you'll be in for the long haul.

What to do after the initial 24-72 hours:

Once the bleeding is controlled, the healing begins. The blood and the damaged cells that have leaked into the surrounding tissue must now be collected through the lymph system and cycled out of the body. At this stage of the healing process, treatment has three primary goals:

- Influence the formation and placement of scar tissue

  - This is the type of tissue the body will use to fill in any damaged tissue area
  - Scar tissue doesn't have a specific pattern and therefore it's placement needs to be influenced by the movement and stress placed on the body part
- Regain full range of motion
  - Be able to move as far in each direction as is normal for that body part and an individuals required performance level
- Reestablish efficient neural pathways of muscle firing
  - The brain develops work arounds when function is interrupted that become habitual the more they are used
  - Retraining muscle patterns to be as efficient as possible at producing the desired movement takes a gradual increase in intensity and consistent practice as the injured area is able to handle it, so the less desirable pattern is replaced by the desired one

This process is best pursued with the help of a physical therapist or a certified athletic trainer. Even just a few visits can provide essential guidance on what to do on your own. Experience has taught me, however, that people are generally not very diligent about pursuing home exercise plans. Many people discontinue treatment once normal performance in everyday activities is restored. Function levels that are adequate for regular activities are not enough for the demands of sports performance. Injuries that are not given enough time to heal, enough rehabilitative effort, or enough support through the remodeling phase will often recur, or drag on unnecessarily. A half-effort during rehab is a primary cause of disappointing post-injury performance, ongoing pain, and immense frustration. Diligent rehab work, by contrast, will help prevent reinjury, speed full recovery, enhance athletic performance, and minimize the total amount of pain and frustration.

Essential things to remember during ongoing treatment:

- Warm up the injured area before hard athletic activity or practice. This can be 5-10 minutes with a heat pack or 10 minutes of gradual warm up exercises before starting.
- Rehabilitation exercises - get help from a physical therapist or certified athletic trainer
- Ibuprofen, an anti-inflammatory, can help with pain and the regulation of inflammation the body experiences during this stage, while performing rehabilitation exercises and returning to activity. Acetaminophen can help with pain, but it is not an anti-inflammatory, so it is not as helpful at this stage.
- Ice after activity - 20 minutes with an ice bag or 10 minutes with immersion in an ice bath.
- Continue to use an ace bandage to help push the swelling out of the injured area and give support until swelling is gone. Note: You can wash ace bandages in the washer, but they will last longer if you allow them to air dry instead of putting them in the dryer.
- Use tape, braces, or sleeves during activity during the extended healing process to give support and avoid reinjury.

WHAT TO USE TO ICE

On first thought, you might think applying an ice bag to an injury wouldn't be too difficult. If you've got a new injury, though, you're going to need a lot of ice. Getting enough ice to use regularly can be a problem. Sometimes, you'll find yourself treating an injury when you're not at home or even close to home - do you wait? Where can you get ice? And by the way, kids don't like ice. They don't want to do it - or they won't leave it on.... Here are all my tips and tricks about ice.

At home:

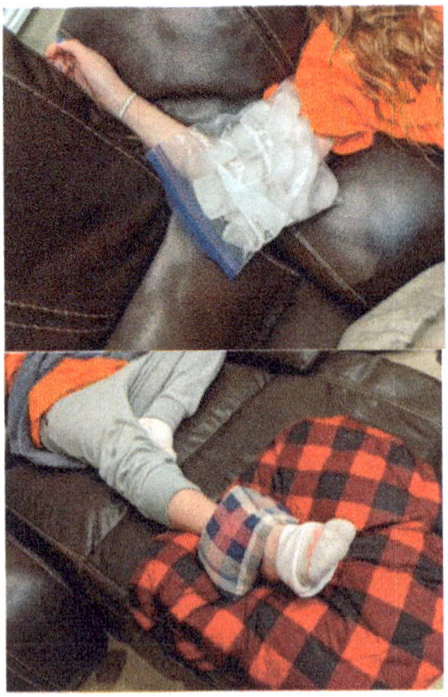

- Put ice from your ice maker in a ziploc bag and store it in your freezer while the ice maker makes more (or your ice trays freeze solid).
- Use a fabric bag with corn or rice inside that you keep in your freezer.
- Use bags of frozen corn or peas - these work really well!
- Use a big bowl or a sink to immerse a hand or foot/ankle in ice water - only use for 10 minutes if you do this!
- Buy a bag of ice at the grocery store, then transfer some smaller amount to a ziploc bag.

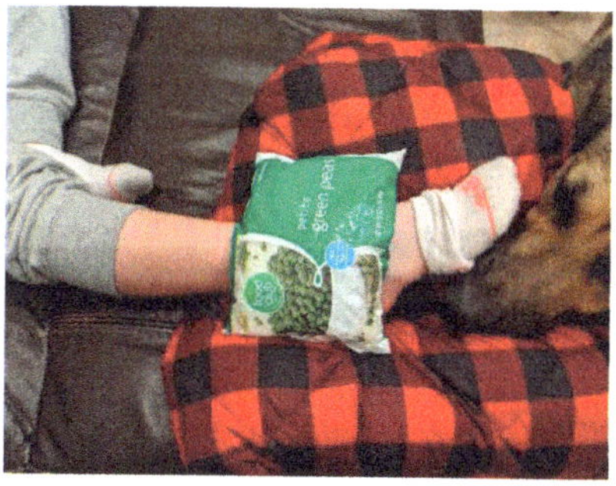

- Keep a reusable gel pack in your freezer. Be aware that this generally won't conform to a body part when it is really cold, so it won't work as well on small areas.
- Freeze paper cups with water in them, then peel the cup down past the ice to rub it on a leg or arm, starting from the end of the extremity and moving up toward the heart. **This method is particularly good for shin splints!**
- Make an ice bath in your bathtub - 10 minutes!
- Sit in a river for 10 minutes.
- Sit in snow in your yard and scoop it up around your legs.

These last few sound kind of crazy, but they're good examples of efficient use of available resources that may be easier and more effective than what you can make work in your bathtub.

When traveling:

- Keep a stash of ziploc bags in the car, and grab some ice at a convenience store or restaurant
- Keep several one time use cold packs in the car. A chemical reaction causes the gel in these packs to get cold, and they last for about 20 minutes.
- If you know you will be using ice for an ongoing problem before you leave home, bring a small cooler with ice in it and some ziploc bags.

Keeping it on:

- I recommend using cling wrap to hold the ice in place
- Younger kids may be better about using a cold bag with corn or rice in it. These don't get as cold as ice bags, but are much more tolerable. If you use this option, put them on more frequently - about 10 minutes on and 30 minutes off.

The power of an ice bath:

While an ice bath is not fun and really difficult to get people to do, those that are brave enough figure out it's amazing, especially for an athlete that is training heavily.

The idea of an ice bath goes back to the theory of patching a hose. When an athlete is working out intensely, they create small tears in their muscles due to both overuse and forceful contractions. Of course this is the process through which muscles grow and strengthen, which is necessary to improve athletic performance, but those tears, though small, can bleed long and slow, and produce soreness and stiffness that lasts day in and day out. There has to be a balance between the strengthening and the soreness, or the level of intense training cannot be maintained. Sitting for 10 minutes in a cold tub helps the muscles to clot off those small bleeders sooner, keeping the soreness from overwhelming the athlete.

- Use a bathtub at home, or in a hotel. Other options include sitting in a nearby river or sitting in the snow in your backyard!
- Buy some ice at a grocery store or keep a running storage of ice from your freezer and dump it into the bath. Put enough in that it doesn't melt immediately.
- Immerse any body parts that are sore.
- Only immerse body parts in an ice bath for 10 minutes. Anything more and body parts could get too cold.
- It is normal to shiver for a while afterward.

Rest assured, they will get used to it after a few times, and won't complain so much!

WHAT TO USE TO HEAT UP

Applying heat to an injured body part brings blood flow into the affected area. The mechanism is this: When you apply heat, your body sends more blood to the surface blood vessels in order to dissipate the heat and regulate body temperature. Once the initial bleeding and damage have been controlled, heat can be helpful because greater blood flow helps to bring healing chemicals in and carry damaged cells out of an injured area.

The increased blood flow triggered by heat also helps structures to be more flexible and stretch without damage that can occur when structures are cold and stiff. During recovery, you'll want to heat an injured area before doing rehabilitation activities, to get the most out of the session. You'll then want to ice afterward, to limit soreness caused by the activities. Whenever a body part is stiff and sore, heat before vigorous activity can improve performance and reduce the risk of injury.

Spending several minutes performing movements that involve many muscle groups, like jogging or biking, then moving into more sports specific movements will warm up muscles to be ready for more intense activity.

For some extra help heating up try the following:

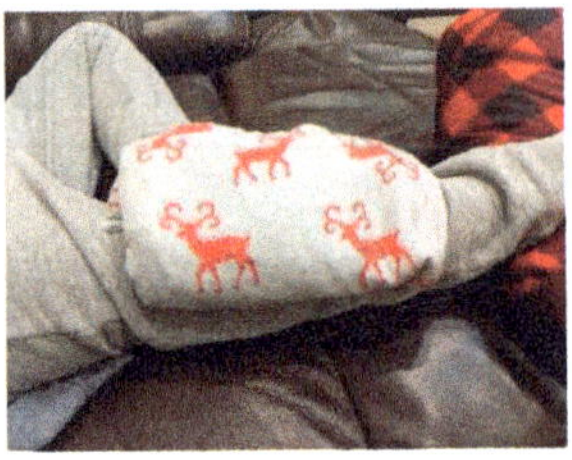

- Heat up a fabric bag of corn or rice in the microwave for 3 or 4 minutes and sit with it on for 8-10 minutes. Try sitting with it in the car to be ready to get going when you get to practice!
- Use a one time use hot pack for 8-10 minutes. A chemical reaction causes the gel contents of the pack to heat up. Be careful with these - they get really hot, so put a layer or two between the gel pack and the skin.
- Immerse the body part in hot water for about 5 minutes.

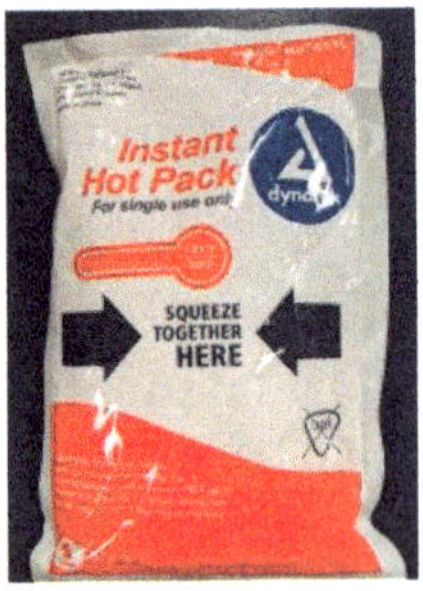

For staying warm while playing:

- Wear a sleeve or shorts made of neoprene or compression fabric directly next to the injured area, under other clothes

- **** PRO TIP****
  Wear a capsaicin patch stuck directly on the skin of the injured area to keep muscles warm. Capsaicin is an herb that comes from chili peppers. The patch provides some serious ongoing heat, and a little pain relief too. Though it feels quite hot, it won't burn the skin. The patches usually come large enough to use on the low back, but they can be cut to any size and used anywhere. My athletes almost always prefer a capsaicin patch to wearing a sleeve. By comparison, sleeves feel bulky on their legs. Capsaicin patches are available online, or at stores that have a pharmacy section.

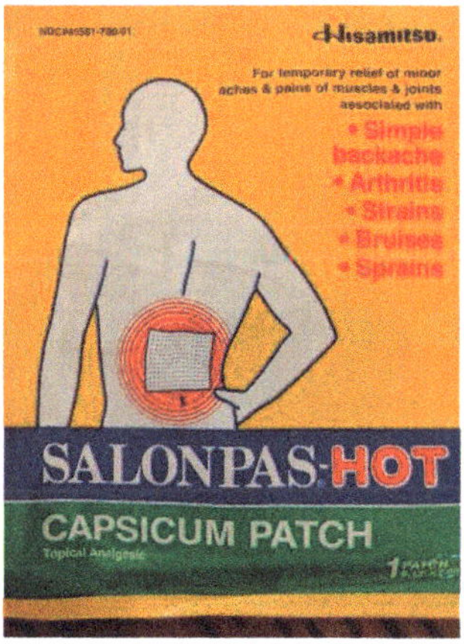
Hisamitsu
For temporary relief of minor
aches & pains of muscles & joints
associated with
• Simple backache
• Arthritis
• Strains
• Bruises
• Sprains
SALONPAS-HOT
CAPSICUM PATCH
Topical Analgesic

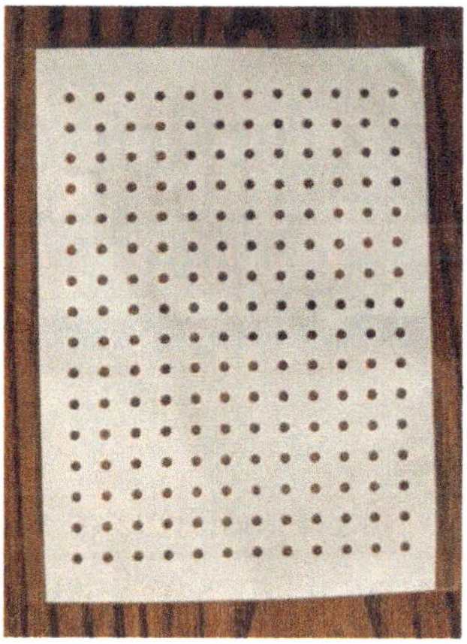

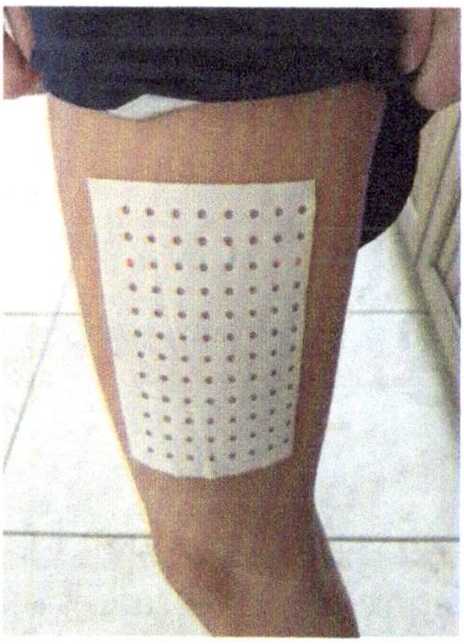

FRACTURES

Fractures are common injuries. It's a good rule of thumb to always suspect a fracture and then rule it out. General types of fractures include compound, displaced, comminuted, non-displaced, avulsion, and stress. In this section I'll explain each of these fractures and what to do about them.

Compound Fractures:

Pieces of bone are poking out through the skin, accompanied by bleeding.

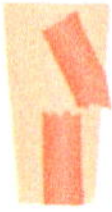

What to do:

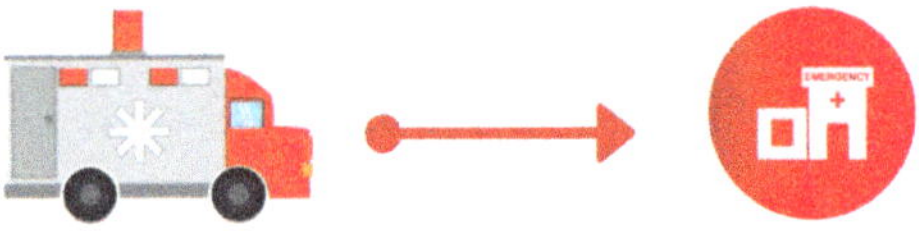

Call an ambulance. Loss of blood can be serious, especially with large bones. Shock will likely be a problem, as well as extreme pain. There will be danger of further damage if you move the body part around.

Obviously Displaced Fracture

Bones sit at odd angles or something just doesn't look right.

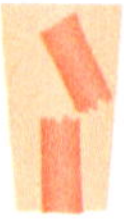

Comminuted Fracture:

The bone is broken into three or more pieces.

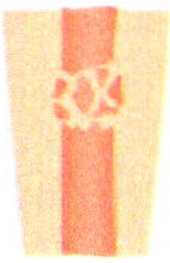

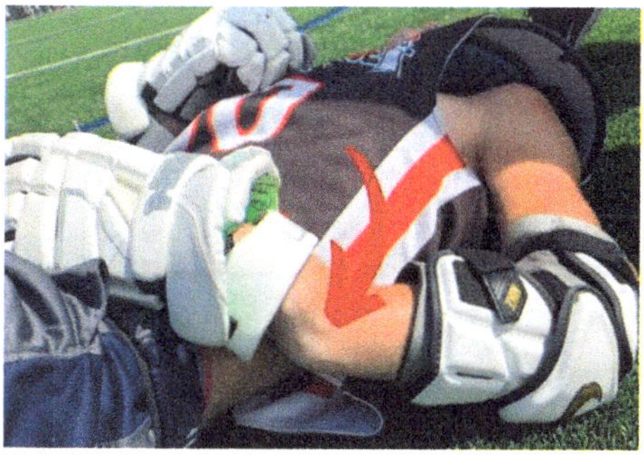

What to do:

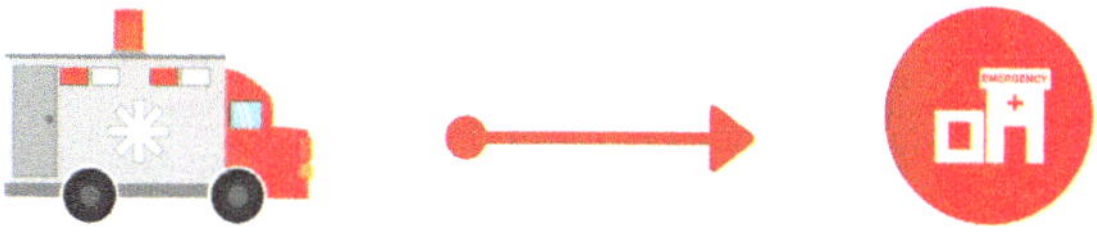

Call an ambulance. Pain will be extreme, and there is risk of further damage if you move the body part around. Shock could also be a problem. Pay attention to blood flow and nerve conduction in the body part below the injury. If the skin is an abnormal color, or there is inability to move fingers or toes, or feel you touch them, structures have been damaged or are being pinched. You don't want to make that worse, and the problem needs to be addressed quickly.

Displaced - but not obvious

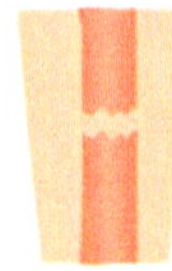

A bone can be displaced, meaning the fragments don't line up nicely because of the position the bone pieces are sitting in, while the bones are still fairly close to each other.

Non-displaced

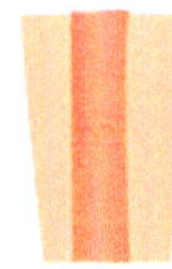

The broken pieces have not moved apart, which makes healing simpler.

Avulsion

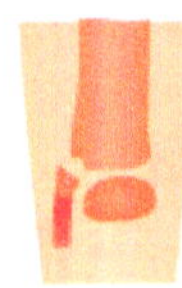

An avulsion fracture is a when a ligament pulls off a small piece of the bone, rather than the ligament tearing.

What to look for when it's not obvious:

There are several signs which should make you suspect there's a fracture:

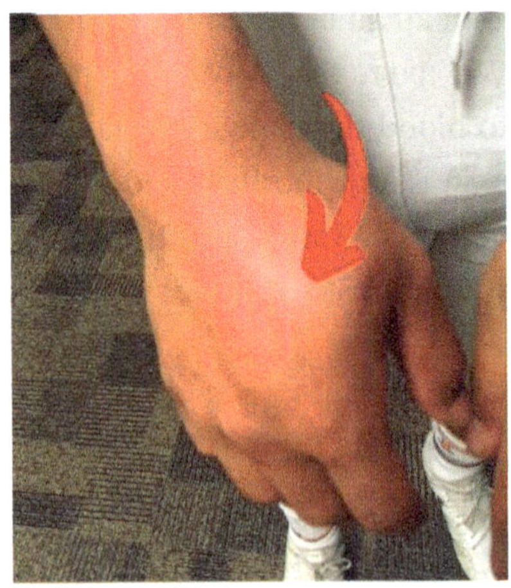

- A large amount of pain
- Motion is severely restricted - compare the injured side to the non-injured side for reference
- Can't bear weight on it (too painful)
- Pain shoots through the surrounding area when the injury site is pressed on
- Swelling
- Bruising

What to do:

In the case of a major amount of pain when just sitting still:

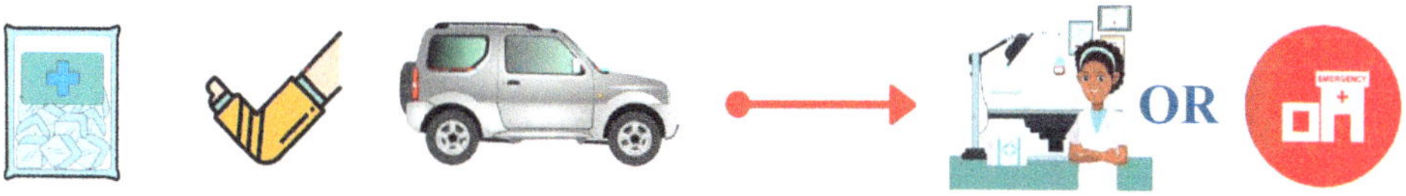

- Ice (20 minutes on and 1.5 hours off)
- Splint above and below the injured area

    - Keep a moldable splint and an ace bandage in the first aid kit in your car. Mold the splint to fit above and below the joint and wrap it on with an ace bandage

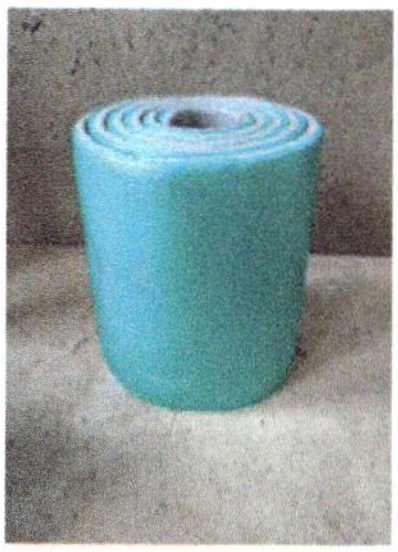
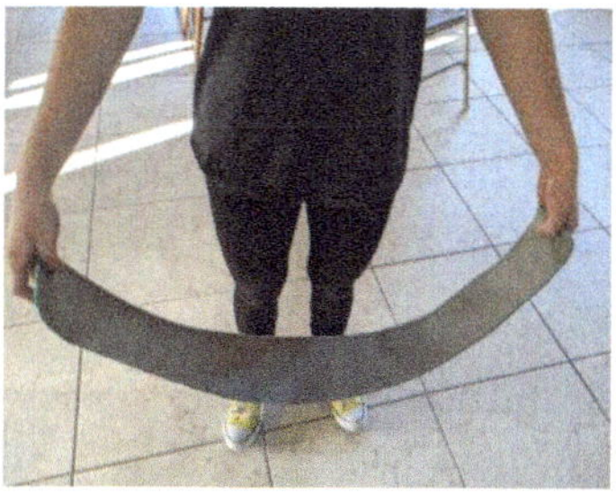
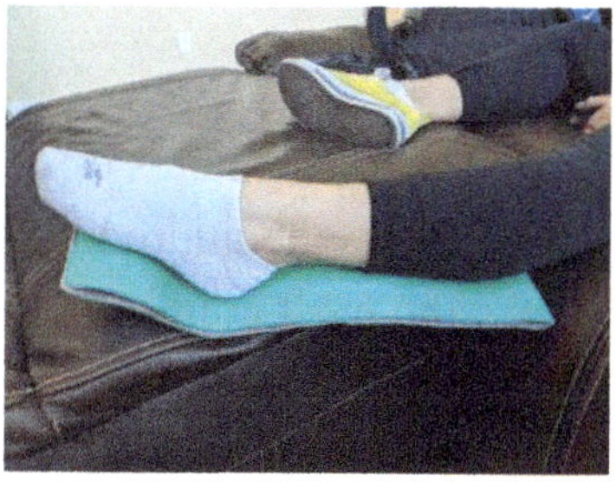
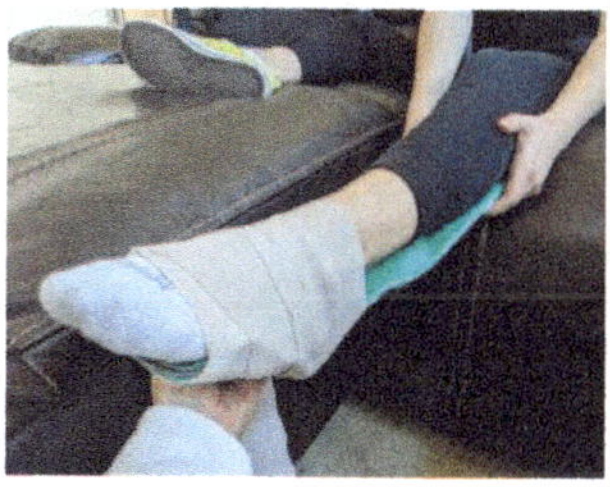
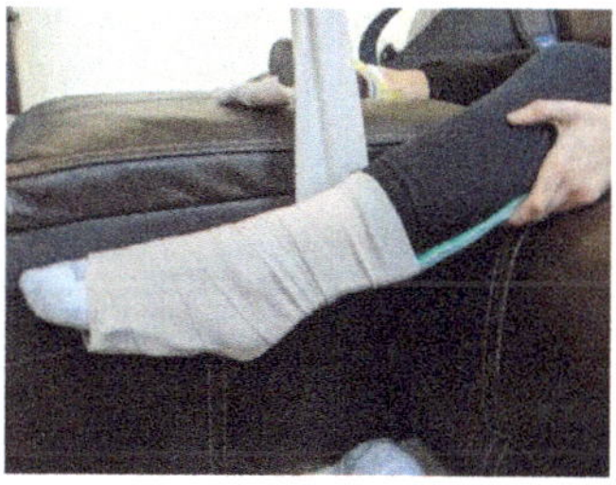
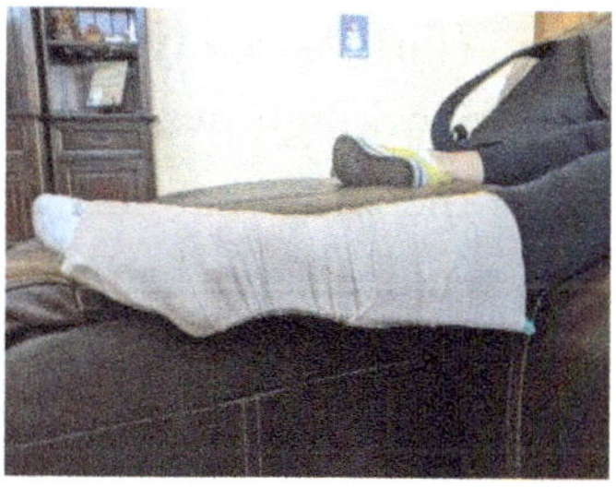

- Elevate the injured body part
- Give acetaminophen for pain - NOT ibuprofen
- Give reassurance, speak positively
- Drive the injured person to a doctors office if you can get in quickly, if not go to the ER

In the case that pain is managed when not moving, and you are not sure if symptoms of fracture are quite there, or they take time to show up:

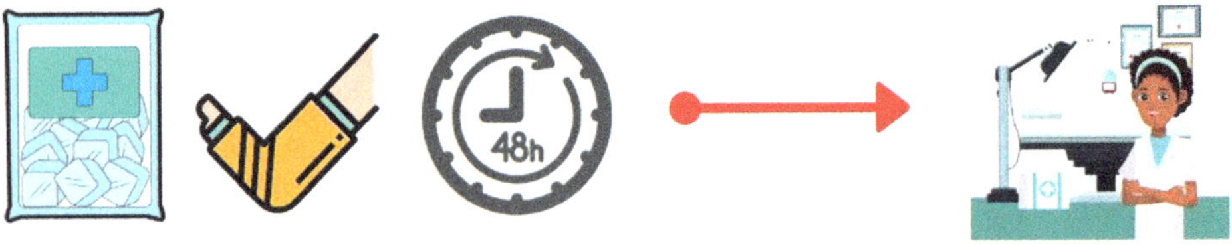

- Ice (20 minutes on and 1.5 hours off) for the first 24-72 hours
- Wrap the injured body part in an ace bandage. Position the body part in the most comfortable position possible. Start wrapping in the extremity below the injured area (furthest away from the heart) and working toward it. Any part of the wrap that goes past the injured area can be loose. Keep the wrap on except while icing, especially at night. The injured body part will tend to throb at night, so it is important to loosen the wrap up a bit to accommodate that, without taking it off completely.

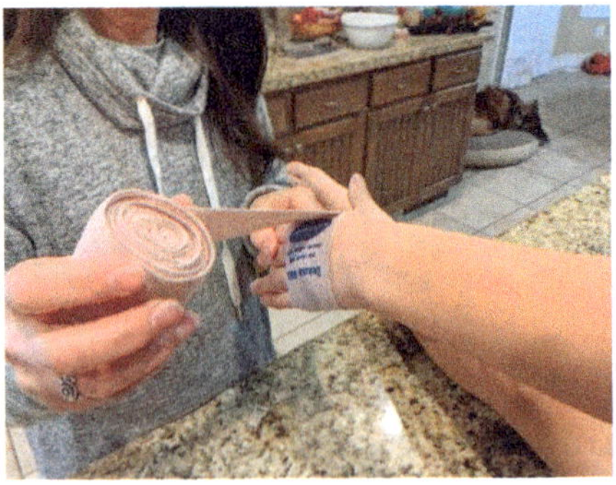

- Give acetaminophen for pain - NOT ibuprofen
- Give reassurance, speak positively

- Watch to see how the injury progresses over the next few days. If pain is not improving, motion is still limited, it swells, and/or it bruises, then you should see a sports medicine physician as soon as you can get an appointment.

Stress Fracture

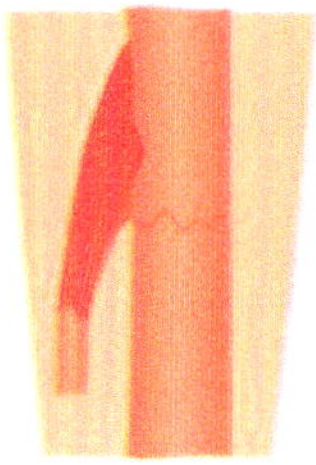

A stress fracture occurs when an area is subjected to overuse, usually with an increase in training levels or amount of time spent in activity. It can also occur with a change in footwear that exposes the body to a different level of force distribution. Young women, particularly, are vulnerable to stress fractures due to hormonal issues, inadequate energy consumption, and lower bone density.

What to do:

Anytime there is pain with no remembered cause of onset, suspect a stress fracture, especially if there has been a shift in the training regiment to a greater intensity or greater amount of training (beginning of a season, moving to a higher level of play, running greater distances). Any female should be seen by a doctor to address the possibility of low bone density, hormonal issues, and/or disordered eating that often are behind stress fractures.

- Ice (20 minutes on and 1.5 hours off) for the first 24-72 hours
- Give acetaminophen for pain - NOT ibuprofen
- Experiment with rest - several days or a week. If pain subsides with rest, but returns when engaging with activity, a stress fracture is a good possibility. Usually, stress fractures will not show up on an x-ray until at least 2 weeks after onset of pain. This is because they are too small to see on an x-ray, and what you are seeing after that much time is the

bone laying down extra calcium in the damaged area. Sometimes, it still won't be visible on a regular x-ray, but a stress "reaction" can be seen on a bone scan. It's not necessarily worth getting a more expensive test so you can "see" it. Treatment will be the same, one way or the other. Treatment will be rest, and depending on where the fracture is located, a boot or some time spent non-weight bearing will be needed.

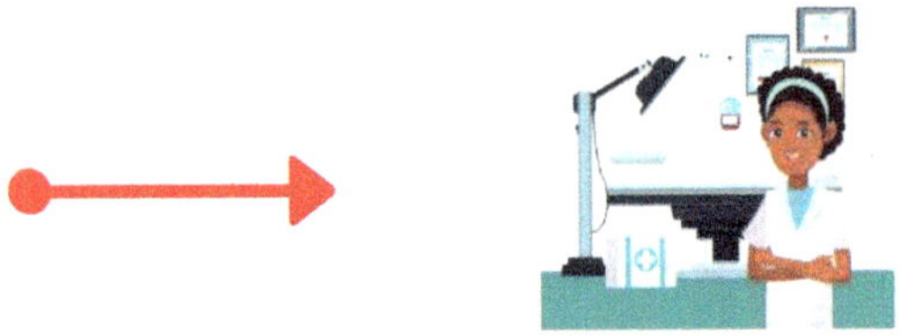

- See a sports medicine physician, after you have tried out giving it some rest, and it continues to be a problem.

Types of fracture illustrations:
Illustration <a href="https://www.dreamstime.com/types-bone-fracture-image186889942">186889942</a> © <a href="https://www.dreamstime.com/vonuk1_info" itemprop="author">Anatoly Shevkunov</a> - <a

DISLOCATIONS

Dislocations happen at joints, where the ends of bones are forced out of their normal position and prevent normal motion. They are extremely painful, and cause damage to the surrounding ligaments, tendons and muscles. The bones themselves can also be fractured in the process.

Dislocations can be emergency situations, if they cause disruption to blood flow and/or nerve conduction.

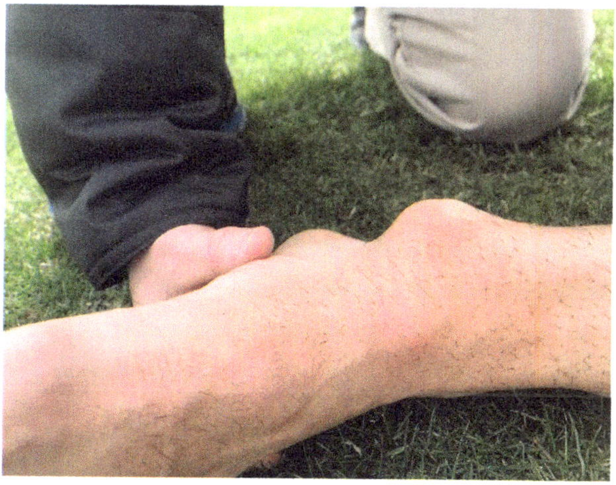

Dislocations stuck out of place need to be put back in by a physician. It is imperative that there is x-ray verification that the bones are completely back in their normal positions. Healing can't proceed until this happens, nor can the damage to other structures be addressed.

Dislocations of knees, hips, and ankles can happen, but they are rare, and when they do, they are a huge emergency! Dislocation at one of these joints means the injury involved a tremendous amount of force and, consequently, a lot of associated damage to surrounding structures. The damage to nerves and/or blood vessels is what creates the emergency.

The most commonly dislocated joints are:

Shoulders, elbows and kneecaps.

Shoulders:

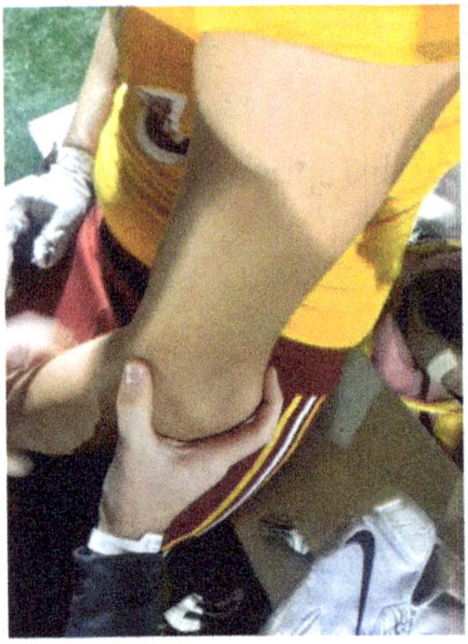

Most commonly, the top of the arm will come out of the joint to the front and sink down, so the ball portion of the arm will be sitting in the armpit. Due to cartilage and ligament stretching or tearing, this can become a recurrent problem, especially when a sport requires overhead movement. This problem can only be solved with surgery. If the initial incident isn't too bad, and is followed by maintained aggressive muscle strengthening and the demands of the sport don't require overhead activity, surgery may be avoided. Seek a sports medicine physician's advice.

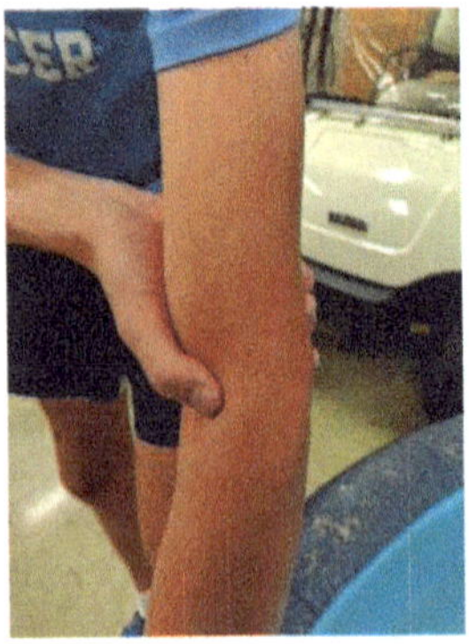

Elbow:

Most often the point of the elbow will be sitting behind where it should be. This injury requires a long rehabilitation effort, in which it is imperative to regain the ability to fully straighten out the arm.

Knee cap:

Most often the bone will be stuck towards the outside of the knee. Due to a structural predisposition for this injury, and the tearing of structures that hold the kneecap in place, this can also become a recurrent problem that can only be solved by surgery. Seek the advice of a sports medicine physician.

What to do for a dislocation:

Problems with circulation and nerve conduction:

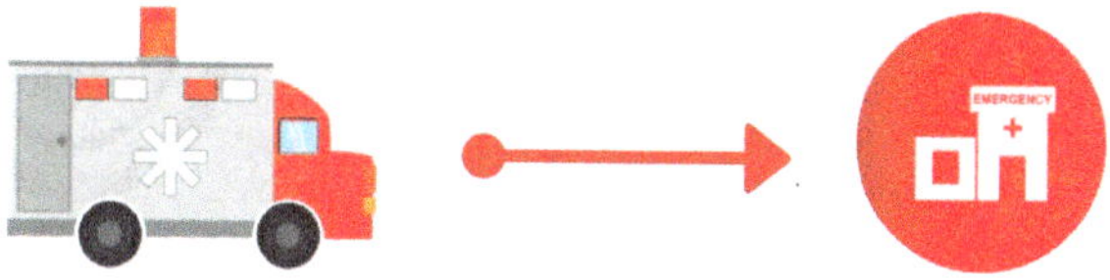

You have an emergency that requires an ambulance if any of the following are true:

- If the body part below the dislocated bone is an abnormal color
- The injured person cannot move the fingers or toes of the associated limb
- The limb has abnormal sensation in it

No circulatory or nerve conduction problems:

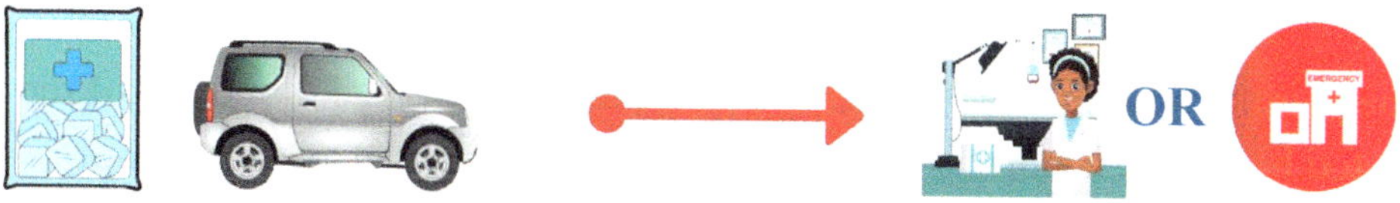

You can drive the person to the ER or straight to the doctors office, if you can get them in quickly. Put some ice on the dislocated body part, prop the limb up with something to limit pain caused by hanging down, avoid moving it around, and go!

Sometimes a bone will shift out of place and quickly pop back in. This is referred to as a subluxation.

What to do:

In the short term:

Rest, ice, compression, elevation.

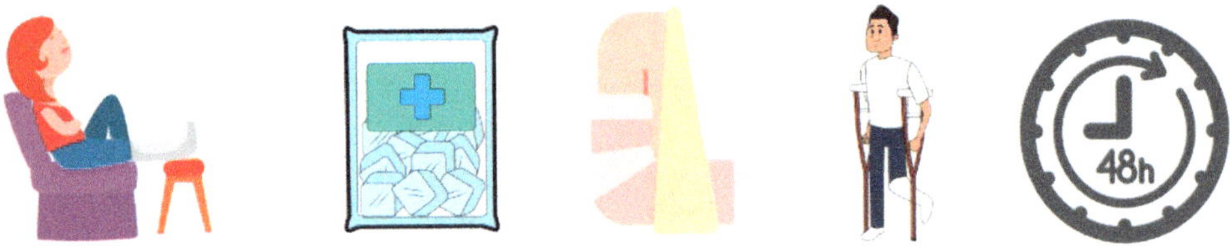

- Rest by not using the body part very much. Use crutches or a sling to take weight off the body part and discourage activity.
- Ice for 20 min, then go 1.5 hours off, and continue as much as you can over the next 24-48 hours
- Wrap the body part with an ace bandage, starting further away from the heart and wrapping towards the heart
- Keep the body part up off the floor, and prop it up when laying down.
- Check for the ability to move the body part, compared to the motion available on the uninjured side, and monitor pain level.

If the pain fades within the first 24 to 48 hours and the range of motion of the affected body part is normal or nearly normal, then you can avoid a doctor visit. The athlete should work on getting full range of motion and engage in a strengthening program with an athletic trainer or a physical therapist, while gradually returning to full sports participation. If the athlete diligently pursues a strengthening program, there will be a good chance of full recovery. Without a strengthening program, however, there is a high probability that the dislocation will recur, and even become a chronic situation.

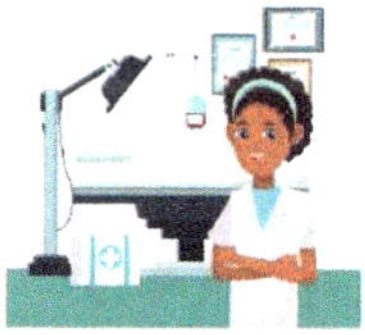

If the range of motion of the affected body part is moderately or significantly restricted and any effort at movement causes pain, see a sports medicine physician ASAP. The physician can help you assess the damage, and make a plan for treatment.

CONCUSSIONS

Concussions occur from a blow to the head. In sports, this usually occurs when athletes knock heads or someone's head collides with part of another athlete's body. It can also happen when an athlete's head hits the ground, floor, or a stationary piece of equipment, or when an athlete is hit in the head by a ball traveling at high speed. Interestingly, concussions can also occur in situations where there is no impact, but a rotational or whiplash motion happens while the body is decelerating.

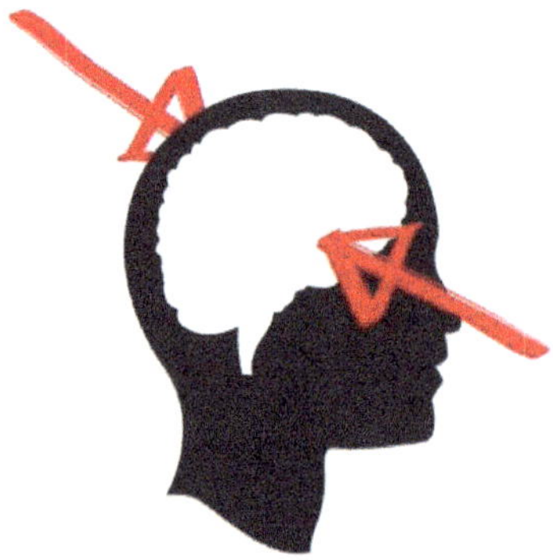

Any of the above listed mechanisms force the brain, which is floating in the head, to slosh in the direction the force pushes it, until it slams into the skull on the side of the head. This abruptly sends the brain sloshing back the way it came, until it slams into the skull on the other side. This cycle perpetuates itself until the force has dissipated.

Damage from this kind of trauma is chemical and metabolic, not structural. MRI's or CT scans tend to show no structural damage. The problem is that the affected brain cells are not getting enough energy to function properly, as their normal chemical processes have been interrupted.

What functions are affected and what symptoms manifest are related to what portions of the brain were involved in the back and forth contact with the hard surface of the skull, and how much force the blow imparted to the brain, therefore determining the amount of back and forth movement that occurred.

Important points to know about concussions:

- A concussion will take longer to heal in a child than an adult with the same severity of injury. One reason for this is that a child's brain is smaller, and therefore has more room to move back and forth inside the skull, causing more damage.
    - Adult: 3-4 days
    - High school age: 10-14 days
    - Junior high age: 2 - 3 weeks
    - Under 12: 4 weeks

- If someone has had a concussion before, another one is easier to get and takes longer to heal.

- The strongest, most consistent predictor of slower recovery is the severity of symptoms during the first day or two.

- Concussion research indicates that youth of high school age are the most vulnerable population for sustaining a concussion.

- A history of mental health problems or migraines **do** appear to create a greater risk of experiencing persistent symptoms after a concussion.

- ADHD and learning disabilities **do not** appear to create a greater risk of experiencing persistent symptoms after a concussion.

- The most common persistent symptoms are headache and sleep disturbances.

- There is **NO** equipment that can completely prevent concussions. Helmets protect the outside of the skull, but have no effect on the brain moving around inside the skull.

- States have different rules about when athletes who have sustained concussions can return to play. Many require a doctor's clearance. You should find out what the rules are where you live.

- If an athlete experiences any sort of blow to the head, they should be pulled out of practice or a game and evaluated for a concussion. **If the athlete has ANY concussion symptoms, they cannot continue to play in that game or practice that day!** Not every blow to the head results in concussion symptoms, but you must be aware that athletes are **VERY** willing to lie, in order to keep playing, especially if it is an important game, so be thorough and willing to take time with the evaluation.

- It is best to evaluate for a concussion away from the emotion of the situation and the distraction of the game, if at all possible.

- Education of athletes ahead of time, about the seriousness of concussions, is essential to help with their willingness to answer truthfully. Your own education - knowing what you're looking for in an evaluation, is also important, so you can recognize a concussion quickly. If an athlete believes that you know what you're looking for with a concussion, they are less likely to think they can get away with lying to you.

How to evaluate whether an athlete has a concussion:

Start with one major question:

Is the athlete unconscious or conscious?

Please understand that losing consciousness does not automatically mean the situation is an emergency, but it is a clear indicator that you need to proceed carefully. You have to first evaluate emergency factors and, in addition to a head injury, you also have to assume there is a neck injury until you can rule it out.

In most situations, the athlete is conscious and can walk off the court or field, which answers a lot of questions for you, but you still need to be aware that the situation could digress quickly. It's absolutely essential to understand that concussion signs and symptoms evolve over time. Consistent watchfulness and repeat evaluation are necessary.

The steps I have outlined for evaluation here are based on the Sport Concussion Assessment Tool (SCAT 5). I emphasize here that your initial assessment using these steps should not replace evaluation by a medical professional. These steps are simply intended to help you access the medical system at a level appropriate for your situation. We'll start with what to do if the athlete is unconscious. If, in your situation, the athlete is conscious, but down on the court or field, skip to page 43. If your athlete is conscious, and has walked off the field or court, skip to page 48.

Athlete is unconscious

Do not move the athlete unless circumstances are dangerous

Do not remove equipment

Check for breathing -
if not breathing, adjust airway and check again
Check heartbeat

Not OK

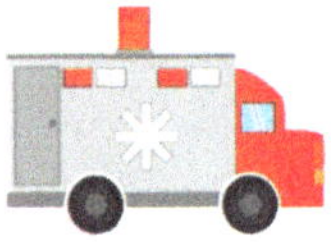

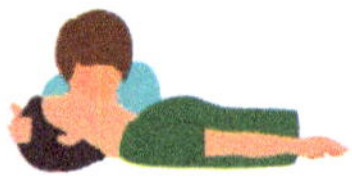

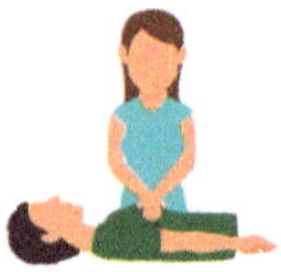

All OK

Jump to the next evaluation box

Athlete is unconscious

Do not move the athlete unless circumstances are dangerous
Do not remove equipment

Check for:

- Seizures
- Convulsions
- Glassy stare - eyes open
- Blood or clear fluid coming from ears, eyes, nose or mouth

Yes to any

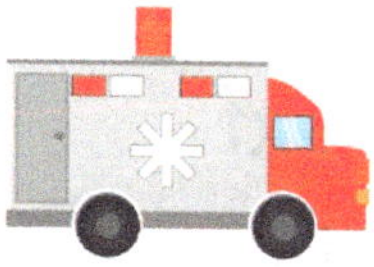

None

Jump to the next evaluation box

Athlete is unconscious

Do not move the athlete unless circumstances are dangerous

Do not remove equipment

Check for the time:

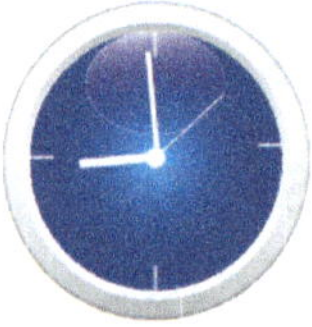

Unconscious longer than 1 min?

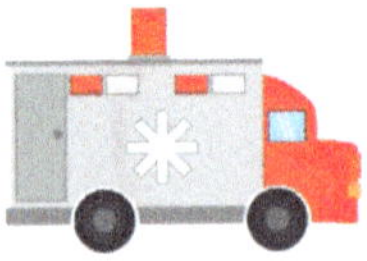

Unconscious less than 1 min

Jump to the next evaluation box

Athlete is conscious but down since injury

Start here

Athlete is conscious

or becomes conscious within 1 min and is down on the court or field

Do not move the athlete
Do not remove equipment

Check the ability to respond

Eyes - open or open when talked to?

Moves according to your command?

Can answer questions?

No to any

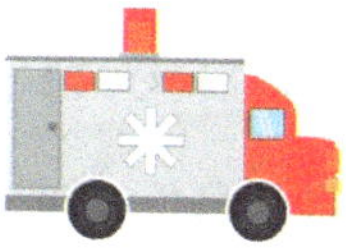

Yes to one or more

Jump to the next evaluation box

Athlete is conscious

or becomes conscious within 1 min and is down on the court or field

Do not move the athlete
Do not remove equipment

Check mental state

Ask questions, such as:
Can you tell me what happened?
What is your name?
Where are you?
What day is it?
Who scored last?

Disoriented and getting worse

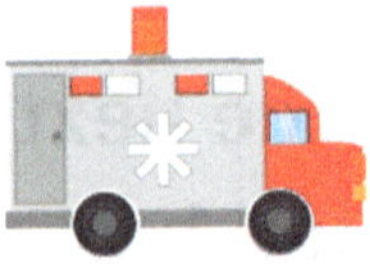

Disoriented but improving or not disoriented

Jump to the next evaluation box

Athlete is conscious

or becomes conscious within 1 min and is down on the court or field

Do not move the athlete
Do not remove equipment

Check for neck injury by asking questions - no neck movement:

- Pain or tenderness on neck bones
- Weakness or tingling/burning in arms or legs
- Any abnormal sensation
- Any of the above come and go

None

Yes to any

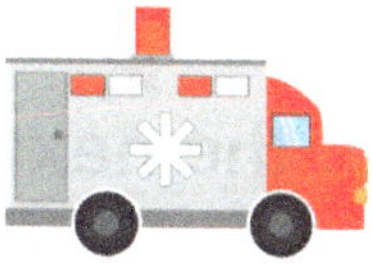

Jump to the next evaluation box

Athlete is conscious

or becomes conscious within 1 min and is down on the field or court

Do not move the athlete
Do not remove equipment

Check neck for pain with muscle contraction - but no movement

Your hand:
On forehead
On one ear
On other ear
On back of head

Athlete:
Pushes into your hand

There is pain and/or abnormal sensation

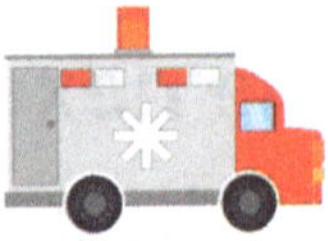

No pain
No abnomral sensation

Jump to the next evaluation box

Athlete is conscious

or becomes conscious within 1 min and is down on the field or court

Do not remove equipment

Check neck with active movement:

Put chin to chest
Tilt head - all the way back
Look to both sides
Tilt head - ear toward shoulder

Full motion
No pain
No abnomral sensation

Move to the sideline and jump to the extreme symptoms evaluation box

There is pain and/or movement causes abnormal sensation

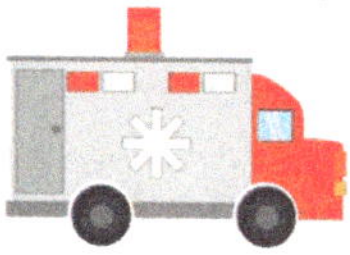

Extreme Symptoms Evaluation Box is on p. 51

Athlete is conscious and walks off the field or court on their own

Start here

Athlete is conscious

or becomes conscious within 1 min and walks off the court or field

Do not remove equipment

Check mental state

Ask questions, such as:
Can you tell me what happened?
What is your name?
Where are you?
What day is it?
Who scored last?

→ **Disoriented and getting worse**

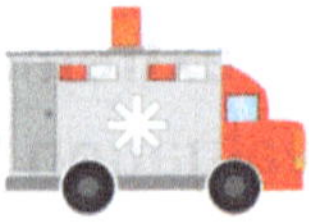

→ **Disoriented but improving or not disoriented**

→ **Jump to the next evaluation box**

Athlete is conscious

or becomes conscious within 1 min and walks off the court or field

Do not remove equipment

Check for neck injury by asking questions - no neck movement:

- Pain or tenderness on neck bones
- Weakness or tingling/burning in arms or legs
- Any abnormal sensation
- Any of the above come and go

Yes to any

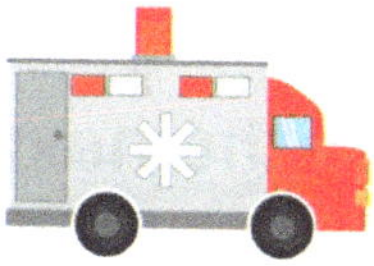

None

Jump to the next evaluation box

Athlete is conscious

or becomes conscious within 1 min and walked off the field or court

Do not remove equipment

Check neck with active movement:

Put chin to chest
Tilt head - all the way back
Look to both sides
Tilt head - ear toward shoulder

There is pain and/or movement causes abnormal sensation

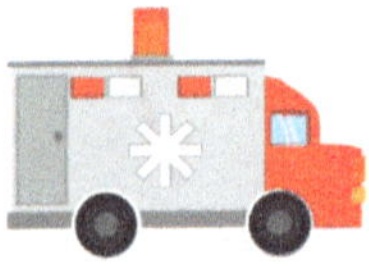

Full motion
No pain
No abnomral sensation

Jump to the next evaluation box

Athlete is conscious

or becomes conscious within 1 min

Remove equipment

Check for extreme symptoms

- Severe or increasing headache
- Double vision
- Vomiting
- Increasingly restless, agitated, or combative

Yes to any

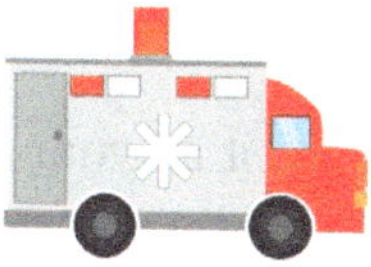

No to all

Move to symptom assessment

If the above extreme symptoms are not present, it's time to evaluate what symptoms there are, and how severe they are.

The list of symptoms is long. In order to document the symptoms, use a spreadsheet to record them. The sample spreadsheet on the next page lists the symptoms and a series of times at which to evaluate. It also asks you to put down a numeric equivalent to the severity of the symptoms. It goes from 0 - 6, with zero being the symptom is not present to 6 being the symptom is extreme. Give it your best guess at first. As time goes on, you'll be able to see which way the symptom is trending.

A copy of the spreadsheet is provided for you to use at the link below in a Google Drive file. Make a copy of it before you start, so you can save it as your private document. While the sample spreadsheet below only goes up to 24 hours, the spreadsheet you will be filling in goes up to 8 days, and you can add more if needed. The P line is for the parent, as you may notice something in the athlete's behavior that the athlete does not. The A line is to enter the number the athlete responds with.

This chart will help you recognize the range of symptoms the athlete is experiencing, and if they are improving, staying the same, or getting worse over time. This information will be good for a doctor to be able to look at, as you work out a treatment and return-to-play plan for the athlete.

Link to Concussion Symptom Assessment Chart:

https://docs.google.com/spreadsheets/d/1gZQHdswKVe0zHjFt5_NfjWvgQ7CPfm3u3ytO4Vvd7uM/edit?usp=sharing

Remember to click File, then make a copy in order to save it as your own Google Drive file.

Concussion Symptom Assessment

Is the symptom present? At what level? Scale = 0-6

0 = not present 1 = mild 2 = mild/moderate

3 = moderate 4 = moderate/severe 5 = severe 6 = extreme

P = Parent's perspective A= Athlete's perspective

Reassess at the given intervals

Symtom	Immediately		15 min		30 min		1 hour		3 hours		5 hours		Next morning		24 hours	
	P	A	P	A	P	A	P	A	P	A	P	A	P	A	P	A
Headache																
Feeling of "pressure in the head"																
Neck pain																
Nausea or vomiting																
Dizzyness																
Memory problems																
Blurred vision																
Seeing stars																
Balance problems																
Sensitivity to light																
Sensitivity to noise																
Ringing in the ears																
Feeling "slowed down"																
Feeling "in a fog"																
"Don't feel right"																
Difficulty concentrating																
Difficulty remembering																
Fatigue or low energy																
Confusion																
Drowsiness																
More emotional																
Irritibility																
Sadness																
Nervous or anxious																
Trouble falling asleep																
Sleep a lot																

The most common concussion symptom and the one that tends to last the longest is headache. A headache can persist for several days, or come and go, depending on what activity the athlete is doing. Trying to concentrate at school or focus on reading or paying attention can bring on a headache long after the initial blow to the head.

After documenting the symptoms, move on to memory assessment. Document this on the second page of the provided spreadsheet.

Athlete is conscious

or becomes conscious within 1 min

Check Immediate Memory and Delayed Recall

Give the athlete 5 words and instruct them to repeat the words back to you in any order, three times in a row:

- Finger
- Penny
- Blanket
- Lemon
- Sugar

Document the number they could remember each time and jump to next evaluation box. After 5 minutes you will ask the athlete to repeat the 5 words again to measure delayed recall. Document the correct number.

After documenting the athlete's ability to remember the immediate memory words, check the athlete's ability to concentrate with the tests below, then ask the athlete to repeat back the words in the above evaluation box to test delayed recall. Document these on page two of the provided spreadsheet.

Athlete is conscious

or becomes conscious within 1 min

Check ability to concentrate

Give the athlete the following strings of numbers - the athlete must repeat them to you backwards

4-9-3

3-8-1-4

6-2-9-7-1

7-1-8-4-6-2

Document if they could do it or not, then move on to asking the athlete to say the months of the year in reverse order

Dec - Nov - Oct - Sep - Aug - Jul - Jun - May - Apr - Mar - Feb - Jan

Document the number correct

In the event an athlete who suffered a blow to the head has no symptoms, and passes all tests:

If an athlete, after a blow to the head, reports no symptoms, has no neck problems, has no balance problems, and can answer all questions appropriately, the next thing to check, before allowing them to go back into the game, is if any symptoms show up with exertion on the sidelines. Increase blood flow to the head by jogging, then running, then quickly changing directions and jumping. If no symptoms show up, then they are good to go!

Make sure the athlete is aware that if they start to get a headache, or any other symptom, they should immediately come out. Getting hit again at such a point, will delay healing, and could seriously increase the damage.

Keep a close watch on the athlete when returning to play.

What to do in the 24-48 hours after an athlete sustains a concussion:

- Keep reevaluating symptoms at the given intervals
- Don't leave the athlete alone
- Taking acetaminophen for headache is okay - but don't give anything stronger
- Have the athlete take usual medication
- Watch for a significant worsening in symptoms or new onset of symptoms
- Make an appointment with a sports medicine physician to address the athlete's situation and make a plan
- Encourage the athlete to stay well hydrated

** The athlete should rest during this time - that means no physical activity, and mental activity should not bring on or worsen symptoms. Reading or focusing on school work can bring on a headache, for example, or the athlete may get more tired after focusing for a while.

Call an ambulance immediately for the following:

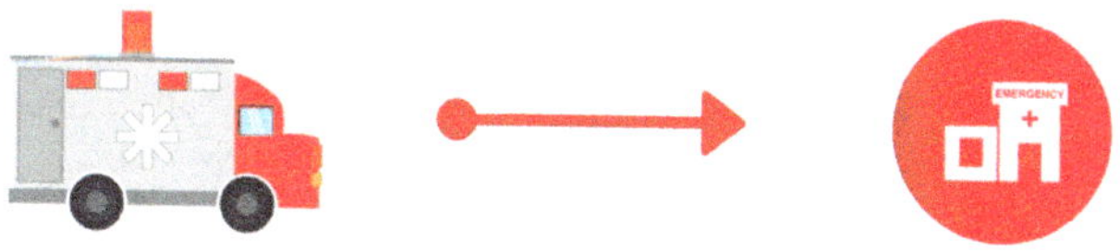

- Seizures
- Decrease in level of consciousness or loss of consciousness

Seek medical care immediately by driving to the ER for the following:

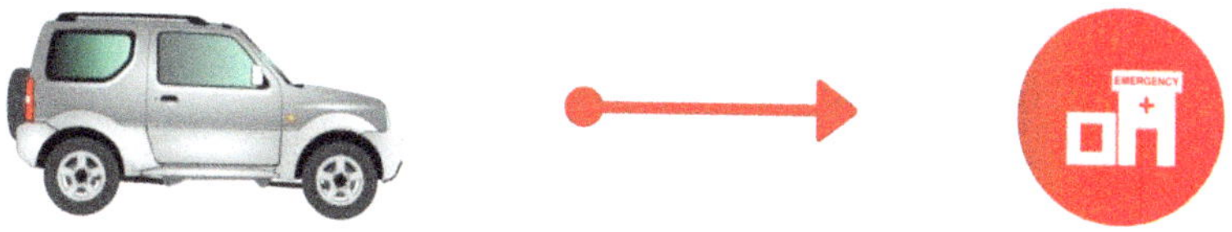

- Significant increase in level of headache
- The athlete is very sleepy and difficult to rouse
- Vomiting
- Any symptoms worsen or new ones show up
- There is anything that seems off about their behavior, that worries you

What a sports medicine physician will want to know at your appointment a few days after sustaining a concussion:

- The list of symptoms the athlete has/had and how they have evolved over time

- Details of any previous head injury
- If the athletes has any learning disability
- If the athlete has ADD/ADHD
- If there are any psychological factors that may influence recovery, such as depression or anxiety
- Academic concerns

What a doctor will help the athlete with:

- Set realistic expectations for a timeline for healing
- Provide guidelines for dealing with symptoms and limiting falling behind at school
- Documentation of the injury for use with school personnel
- Monitoring of symptoms that may be taking an extended time to resolve and referral for further treatment if needed
- A return-to-play progression timeline
- Documentation of final clearance to return to play

What to do when 24-48 hours have passed and the athlete is improving:

This will vary depending on each athlete's particular situation and what symptoms are present. The key is to progressively become more active, while staying below a threshold of symptom aggravation. The athlete needs to self-monitor. If an activity brings on symptoms or makes existing symptoms worse, then they need to try adjusting the activity. If adjusting the activity does not help, they need to stop the activity.

Here are some examples of activity adjustment:

- If computer use is aggravating symptoms, try switching to a different computer. Sometimes a different screen or a larger screen has a different effect.
- Switch to reading a physical book, rather than reading a screen.
- Try a different amount of light.
- Change the spot from which something is being viewed - get closer, get farther, sit so you hold your head in a different position.
- Spend a few minutes on one subject, then switch to another that requires a different type of activity.
- Move in a straight line, as opposed to changing directions.

What a doctor evaluates before clearing an athlete to return to play after a concussion:

- All symptoms are gone - athletes must feel and act completely normal, not just better, or pretty good. The doctor will look in detail at an athlete's general medical history and concussion symptom history.
- A normal neurological exam - includes assessment that all nerves in the head are working properly, hand-eye coordination is normal and balance is normal.
- Neurocognitive function has returned to baseline, if the athlete has completed a baseline test prior to injury, or is within normal limits for their age. This includes verbal and visual memory tasks, both short term and long term. It also includes assessing how quickly the brain processes information and reaction time.
- Follow an organized return to activity progression - this includes a gradual increase in intensity of activity and amount of head movement over a period of days, with monitoring of symptom recurrence at any stage. Make sure the athlete understands that lying about symptoms and moving through this process more quickly than their symptoms allow is quite dangerous and will definitely cause healing time to take longer than it will otherwise.

Return to activity progression:

Below is an example of a return-to-play protocol. Start this when a doctor says the athlete is ready for it. Sometimes this is a few days after sustaining a concussion, and sometimes it can be several weeks. If the athlete tries to do it too early, symptoms will flare up.

First:

- Try a mild activity like riding a stationary bike or a brisk walk for about 15 minutes. The idea is to get the heart rate up without moving the head around very much. This is best accomplished in an environment that doesn't require the athlete to pay much attention to surroundings. **If** any symptoms show up while doing the activity, **stop** the activity and wait a few more days before trying again. Also watch for any symptoms to show up in the hours after doing the activity, and if they do, then wait a few more days.

If the mild activity did not bring on any symptoms, then:

- **The next day**, try a more intense activity like running and some sports specific skills for 20-30 minutes. This may involve a ball and other equipment the athlete normally uses. This could also involve resistance training. The point is to increase the level and duration of exercise, and introduce more coordinated movements. **If** any symptoms show up while doing the activity, **stop** the activity, and wait a few more days before trying again. It is okay to go back down to the mild activity level in between. If symptoms show up within a few hours of the activity, that also disqualifies the athlete from moving on.

If the more intense activity did not bring on any symptoms, then:

- **The next day**, the athlete can return to noncontact training. This includes sports specific complex drills that can involve quick changes of direction and jumping. **If** any symptoms show up while playing, **stop** playing at that level. Reduce the level of activity, wait a few more days, then try again. If any symptoms show up in the hours just following non-contact training, the athlete is not ready to move on.

If no symptoms arise with noncontact training, then:

- **The next day**, the athlete will be able to return to full contact play. Just as with other days in the progression, **if** any symptoms show up while playing, **stop** playing at that level. Return to a lower level of activity and wait a few more days before trying again. If any symptoms show up later in the day after full contact training, the athlete is not ready for a full game situation yet.

If no symptoms arise with full contact training, then:

- **The next day**, the athlete can return to game play. Many states require a doctor's clearance in written form for the athlete to return to play.

Sources:

SCAT 5

SCAT 5 Child

International Consensus Statement on Concussion in Sport

Medbridge Education, Concussion in Sport Parts 1 and 2, presented by Dr. Todd Arnold

COMMON SHOULDER INJURIES

AC Joint Sprains (often referred to as an AC separation)

This occurs where the collar bone connects to the shoulder. There are 3 degrees of this injury.

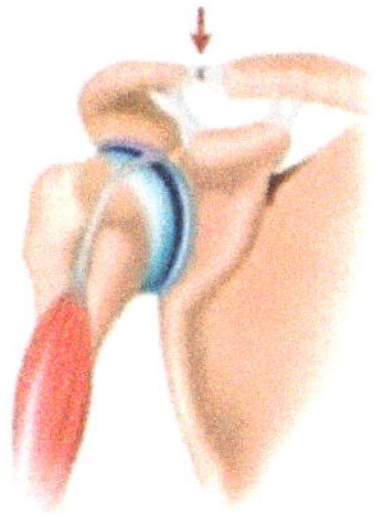

Grade I

First degree: Minimal damage, so there will be pain at the joint site and some limitation to motion, but no obvious deformity. Moving the arm from straight out across the front of the body will be especially painful.

What to do:

- Ice - 20 min on, 1.5 hours off for the first 24-48 hours
- Wearing a sling can help ease the pain associated with the arm hanging down
- Use acetaminophen NOT ibuprofen for pain
- See a sports medicine physician within a few days time

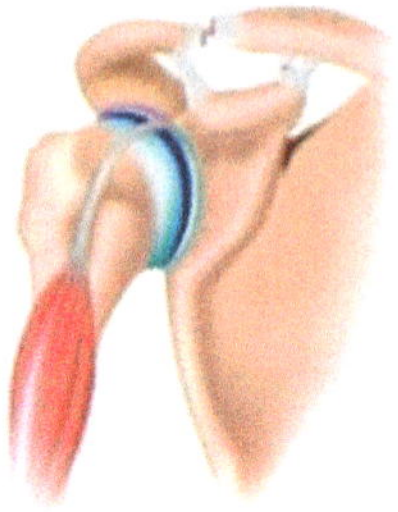

Grade II

Second degree: The collar bone will be sitting a little higher on the injured side, so you will see it poking up. There is a significant amount of pain and lack of motion associated. Moving the arm from straight out across the front of the body will be especially painful and limited.

What to do:

- Ice - 20 min on, 1.5 hours off for the first 24-48 hours
- Wear a sling
- Use acetaminophen for pain, NOT ibuprofen
- See a sports medicine physician ASAP

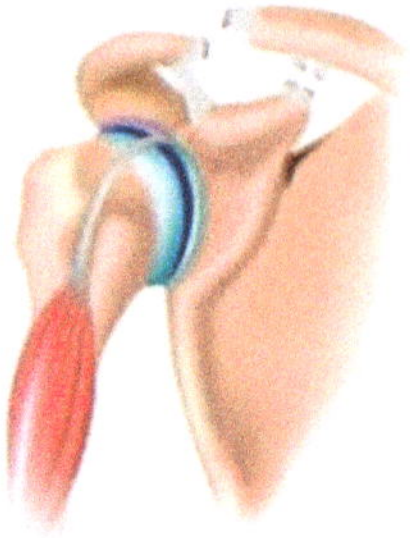

Grade III

Third degree: Several structures are torn, so the collar bone will be poking up a lot higher on the injured side. Pain is intense and motion severely limited, especially moving the arm from straight out to across the front of the body.

What to do:

- Ice - 20 min on, 1.5 hours off for the first 24-72 hours
- Wear a sling
- Use acetaminophen for pain, NOT ibuprofen (Prescription pain medication is really helpful with the injury, because sleeping is especially difficult)

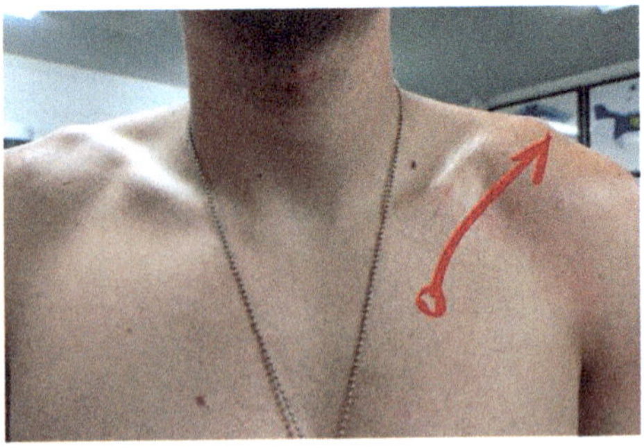

- See a sports medicine physician ASAP. Surgery is an option for this injury, but not an absolute must. It depends a lot on what activities the athlete engages in. This injury can heal on its own, but the collar bone will always sit higher up than normal

Illustrations 28181333 © Alila07 | Dreamstime.com

Dislocation:

The top of the arm most commonly will dislocate to the front, and sink down into the armpit area. It will look obviously deformed, and cause a lot of pain. It can dislocate to the back, but the shoulder blade is there, so that is not as common. Any complete dislocation that stays out of place can cause damage to ligaments, cartilage, tendons and the joint capsule. Sometimes bones will be fractured as well. The dislocated bone can rest and put pressure on structures it normally wouldn't, causing disruption of blood flow or nerve function. A doctor needs to put the shoulder back in place ASAP. The doctor will also need to ascertain through x-ray that it is in place correctly and that there are no associated fractures. The severe pain will ease as soon as the bone is popped back into place, but aching from damaged structures will persist.

What to do for a complete dislocation that stays out of place:

A dislocation accompanied by problems with circulation and nerve conduction:

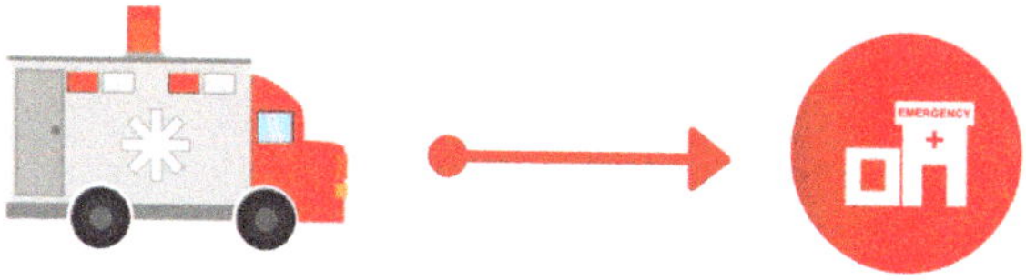

If any of the following are true, they indicate circulatory or nerve conduction problems and you need to call an ambulance:

- the arm below the dislocated bone is an abnormal color
- the athlete cannot move their fingers
- the arm has abnormal sensation

A dislocation with no circulatory or nerve conduction problems:

Ice and go!

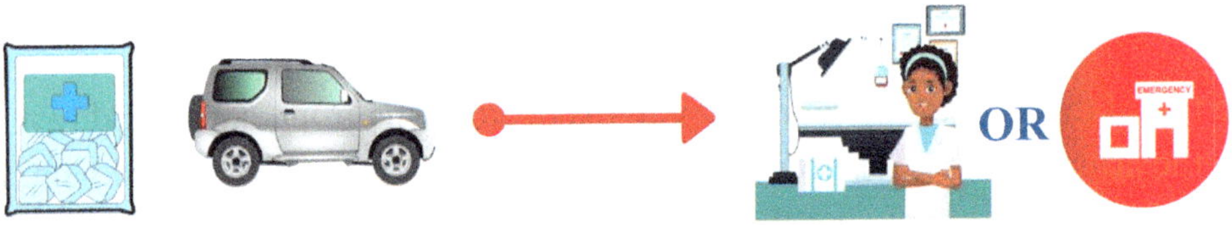

You can drive the person straight to the doctors office, if you can get them in quickly or to the ER if not. Put some ice on the dislocated body part. Prop the arm up with something to limit pain caused by the dislocated part hanging down and to avoid having it cause more damage by moving around, and then go!

After a dislocation, you must expect the athlete to follow a rehabilitation program with a physical therapist or an athletic trainer, in order to strengthen surrounding muscles to help stabilize the shoulder joint. The torn or stretched out ligaments will not be able to keep it in place. This can easily turn into a chronic problem. If it does, surgery will be required to solve the problem.

What to do with a shoulder that pops partially out of place, then quickly back in:

For the first 24-48 hours:

Rest, ice, compression, elevation.

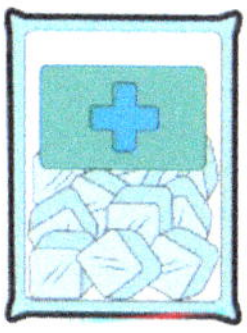

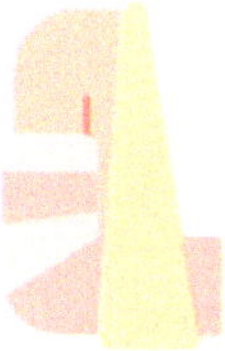

- Rest by not using the arm very much. Use a sling to keep it from hanging down when the athlete is up and moving around.
- Ice for 20 min, then go 1.5 hours off, and continue as much as you can over the next 24-48 hours
- Keep the arm in the most comfortable position possible when sitting and laying down.

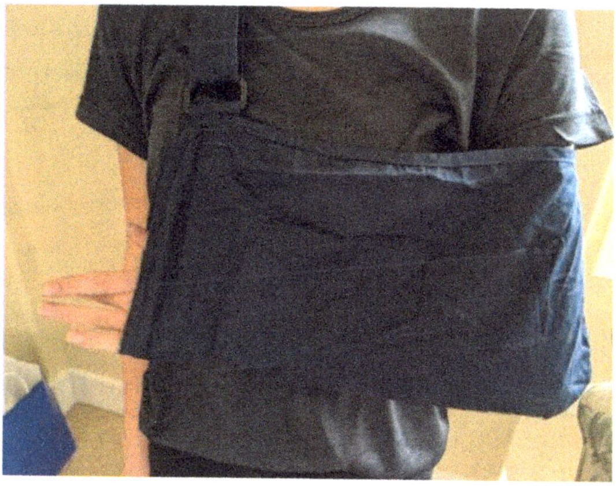

- Check the ability to move it through a normal range of motion and monitor pain level.

If, after 24-48 hours, there is improvement in pain and they are only lacking a small amount of range of motion as they move their arm straight up in front and straight out to the side, then you can avoid a doctor visit. Compare the amount of motion they have with the uninjured side. Work on getting full range of motion and engage in a strengthening program with an athletic trainer or a physical therapist, while gradually returning to full sports participation. If a strengthening program is not pursued, it is a good possibility that it will happen again, and become a chronically recurring situation.

After 24-48 hours:

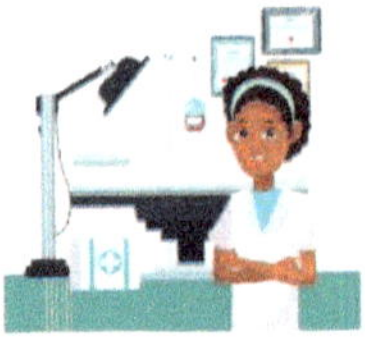

If there is a moderate to significant lack of range of motion and pain associated with any effort at movement, see a sports medicine physician ASAP, in order to assess the damage, and make a plan for treatment.

Impingement:

This is an overuse problem. Inflammation occurs where the tendons pass through the space between the tip of the shoulder and the top of the arm, which causes the tendons to get pinched by the bone, especially during overhead movements of the shoulder.

What to do:

- Stop the activity causing the problem for a week or two to allow things to calm down
- Ice after activity
- Roll out the upper back and front and back sides of the chest and shoulder with a small hard rubber ball.

LOW BACK, HAMSTRING, IT BAND, GROIN AND HIP FLEXOR MUSCLE INJURIES

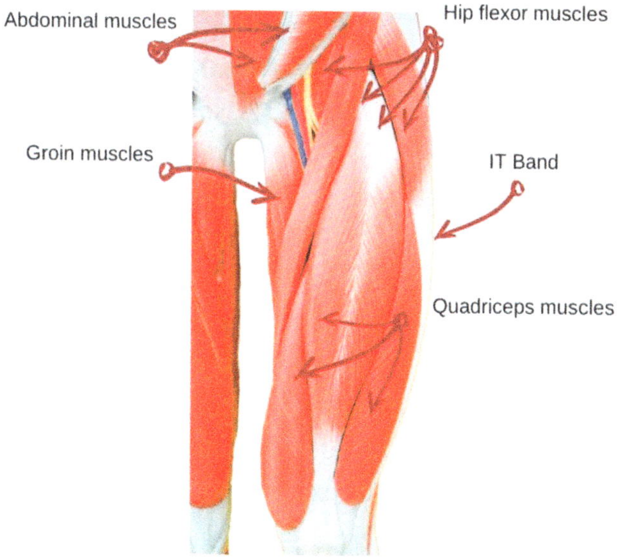

It is really common to have some pain or tightness in the low back, groin, hamstring, IT Band, or hip flexor muscles. The hip, pelvis and lower back transfer force from the lower body through to the upper body, and their position relative to each other shifts constantly due to forces encountered.

Playing sports requires movement patterns that are performed over and over again, and just as you have a hand/arm that is dominant, you have a leg that is dominant. The muscles on the dominant side tend to get tight and irritated from

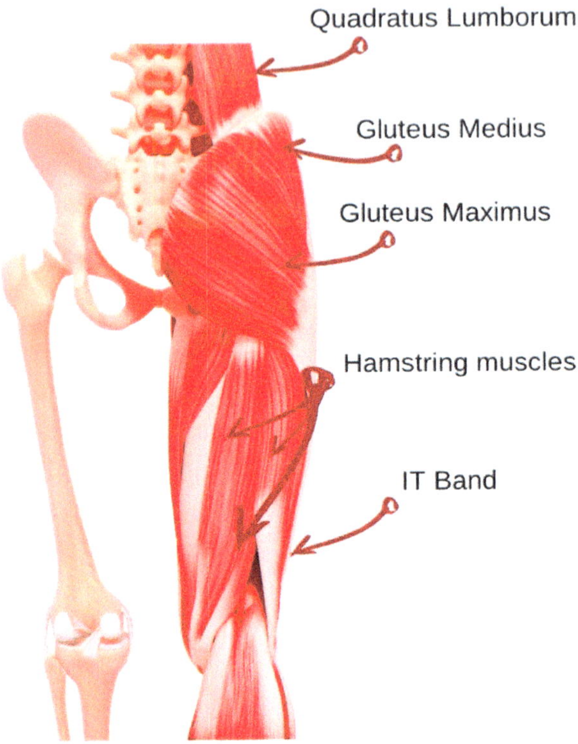

overuse while performing repetitive motions, and the muscles on the other side get tight and irritated from working to stabilize the body while the opposite limb is in motion. This causes the bones to get pulled a bit out of their ideal approximation. Associated muscles, tendons and ligaments end up in either a a longer or shorter than normal position, and movements become less efficient. The pattern described here is one of the most common causes for stretching and tearing in lower body muscles, ligaments and tendons. Stretching and tearing can come from both consistent lower level force exposure or a sudden high level force generation.

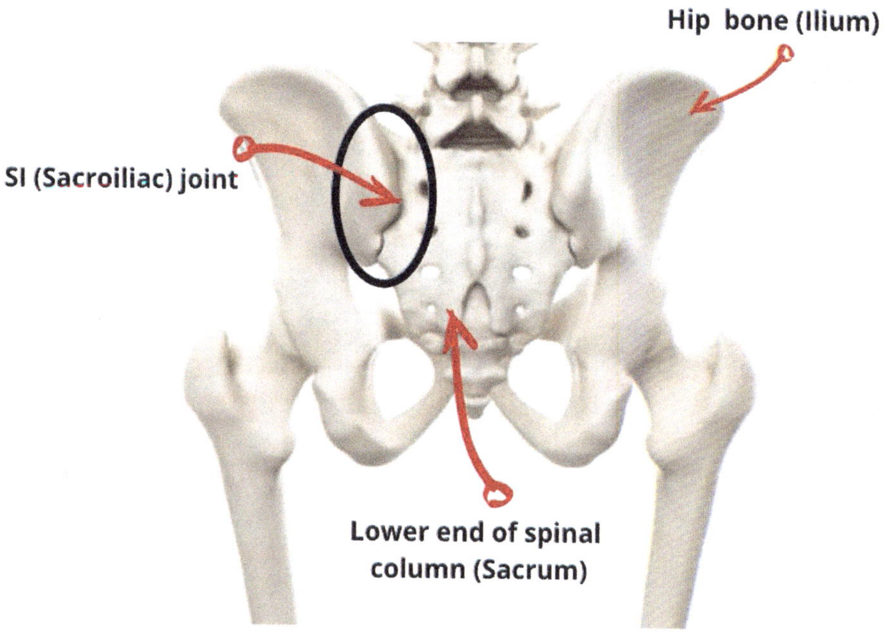

(Illustration 58830906 © Sebastian Kaulitzki | Dreamstime.com)

Most hamstring, groin, IT band, hip flexor and low back problems come about because of the position of the hip bone/s, relative to the lower spinal column. If a hip bone is rotated and/or flared in one direction, the bones of the spinal column will turn sideways or tilt a certain way to compensate. The joint between the sacrum (the end of the spinal column) and the Ilium (part of the pelvis) is called the “SI” joint. This joint can get “locked up”, meaning the bones do not slide on one another as they should. They are stuck together instead and move as a unit. Which other structures are affected by this and how, depends on the position the bones are stuck in. Bones can have more than one positional issue, creating pain and dysfunction in multiple structures. It is also possible for both SI joints to be “locked up” and dysfunctional, creating a lot of low back pain.

The photo below illustrates what I am talking about.
(Photo 14111626 © Skyhawk911 | Dreamstime.com)

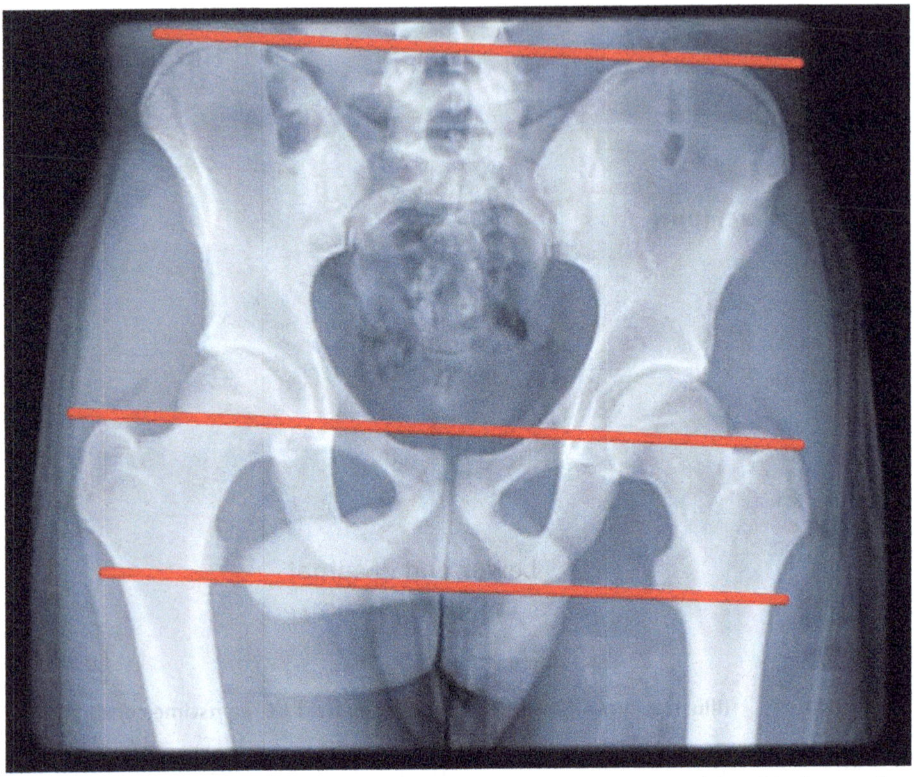

This can all get rather complicated, but the most important bit of information to understand is this: just resting until the affected muscle feels better does not solve the underlying problem. Unless the underlying problem is addressed the irritation will return as soon as the athlete returns to play. Athletes can end up with chronic problems because of hip alignment issues I've described here. I encounter many athletes that come to my team having experienced years of pain and irritation that comes and goes, and has kept them from playing up to their full potential.

So, when an athlete is experiencing persistent lower body pain and irritation, how can you determine whether pelvic alignment is at the root of the problem? Here are some basic things you can check to find out:

One indicator of a hip alignment problem is that one leg will look longer than the other one. To check for this, have the athlete lie down on their back with

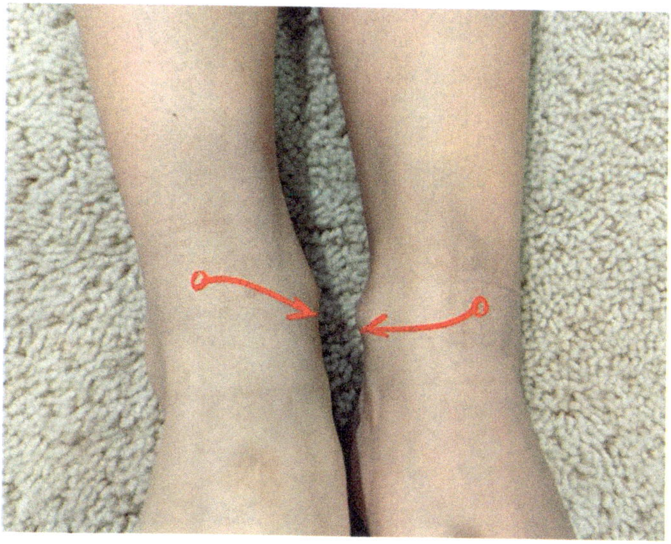

their legs close together. Put your thumbs under the ankle bones on the inside of the legs where the arrows are in the photo below, and look at how level your thumbs are with each other.

As a side note, it is possible, though not particularly common, for one leg to **actually** be longer than the other one. If that is the case, the athlete will definitely have recurring pain. A situation where one leg is actually longer than the other needs to be addressed with a custom-fit lift orthotic in the shoes and you'll need to work with a sports medicine physician to get one of those. Most people, however, don't have one leg that is truly longer than the other, so if one leg is sitting longer than the other one, you can assume a problem with hip alignment.

Another way you can tell if the hips are out of alignment is by putting your index finger along the top of the hip bone on each side and checking if one is higher than the other. It can help to have someone else do it so you can stand back and look from further away.

The difference may not seem super obvious, but only a small amount of misalignment can be the cause of significant problems.

To treat a hip/SI joint alignment problem, you need to address two different problems: First, you need to take care of the muscle/s that are irritated or injured. Second, you need to get the pelvic bones/SI joint alignment back to a better functional position.

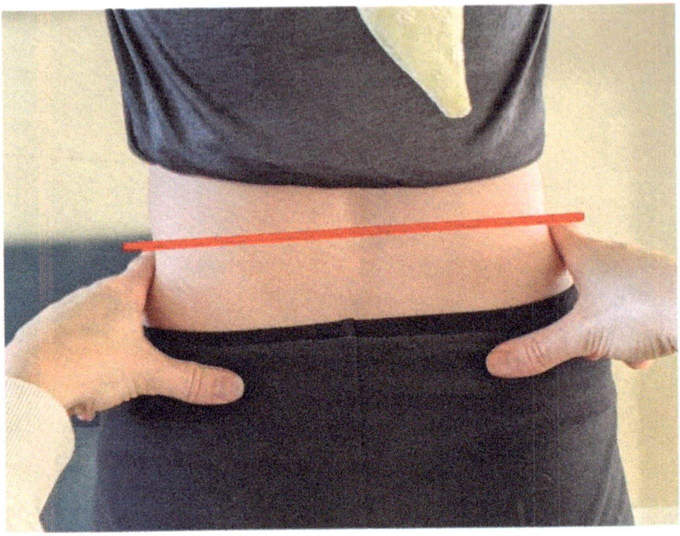

In the event of any injury to the low back, hamstring, IT band, groin, or hip flexor muscles:

First, do damage control for 24-72 hours, depending on the severity.

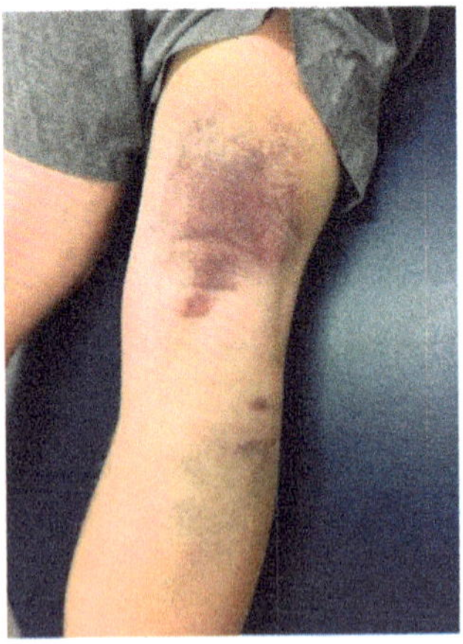

Mild injury = tightness, discomfort, soreness, pain that equates to a 1-3 or 4 on a 10 point scale. The athlete may limp, but can still bear weight and get around. You might see some bruising showing up after a day or two.

Moderate to severe injury = pain of a 4 to 8 on a 10 point scale. Difficulty bearing weight and moving at all. Expect bruising that can be deep colored and extensive.

Severe injury = pain reported as an 8 or above on a 10 point scale. Cannot bear weight, cannot contract the muscle or move the leg. Major bruising. If a section of the muscle has been completely torn, it may roll up and look as if a small ball is sitting under the skin.

For the first 24-72 hours:

- Rest - Limit physical activity. For pain levels higher than a 3-4 use crutches
- Ice - 20 minutes on, 1.5 hours off as often as you can
- Compression - do this with an ace bandage, a sleeve, or compression shorts. This is super important, especially with moderate to severe injury.
- Elevation - keep legs up by resting them on a chair or something of similar height when sitting down. Prop the injured leg up on something while laying down.
- Use acetaminophen for pain, NOT ibuprofen
- For injuries with pain levels higher than 3-4, that don't improve greatly in the first 24 hours, see a sports medicine physician ASAP and keep following the RICE protocol. As things calm down, and pain is limited and movement restored, find someone to deal with the hip alignment problem and rehabilitation of the muscle.
- For mild injuries that improve quickly, you still need to find someone to work on the hip alignment problem and help with the rehabilitation of the muscle.

Providers who can help you treat a hip alignment/SI joint problem:

The following is important to know about the care different kinds of providers can give:

- A physician that is a DO (Doctor of Osteopathy), but not an MD (Medical Doctor) will be able to help correct pelvic alignment problems. As part of their medical school training, DO's learn what are called manipulations. These are treatment procedures which strategically shift the positions of bones. When you find a DO, be sure to check whether they actively do manipulations in their practice. Some DOs do not. If you look for a DO that specializes in sports medicine or orthopedics they will be more likely to do manipulations. After getting treatment from a DO, you will still need rehabilitation to help with healing and reduce future problems. The DO will probably refer you along to a physical therapist for this treatment.

- A Physical Therapist (PT) will approach pelvic alignment problems in a different way than a DO. All physical therapists can provide care for the actual muscular injury, and rehabilitation through strengthening the injured muscle as well as those in the surrounding area. Not all of them will specifically address hip alignment problems. You will have the best experience if you look for one that regularly works with sports injuries.
- A certified athletic trainer (ATC), like a physical therapist will provide care for the muscle injury and rehabilitation of all related muscles. Not all certified athletic trainers will be trained to directly address hip alignment problems. If you find an athletic trainer you want to work with ask if they know how to do muscle energy techniques for the hip/low back.
- A chiropractor can partially address a hip alignment problem by adjusting the position of the sacrum (the bottom portion of the spinal column). Most chiropractors do not adjust the position of the pelvic bones in relation to the sacrum. Chiropractors also generally don't perform care for the muscular injury, so you will likely have to go to someone else for that.

Crucial aspects of treating a hip alignment/SI joint problem and avoiding the build up of one going forward:

Even if bones get put back into place, if surrounding muscles are still tight, they will be pulled back out of place rather quickly. And if the bones are out of place, the muscles will get irritated. This is an ongoing cycle that is only broken by loosening up the muscles and relieving inflammation. While seeking help from a professional is necessary here, there are things you can do at home to help speed the process up, and consistently do to avoid significant problems in the future:

- Massage - Any painful spots that are harder than surrounding muscle are called "knots" and are the problem you are looking for. Knots are areas of chemical imbalance within the muscle where a portion of the muscle stays partially contracted, usually to protect an injured area. These have got to be broken up, restoring normal patterns of muscle contraction and bringing in blood flow. Massage here is not pleasant, but the injured area will feel so much better afterward, that it's worth it!

  Options for massage:
    - Rub by hand, using lotion or some kind of oil
    - Roll on a softball or lacrosse ball for buttock muscles. Roll with the ball against the wall. Deep buttock pain is common while doing this - but it's necessary!
    - Use a firm roller for quads, IT Band, groin and calf muscles. Generally speaking, roll onto a painful spot, then hold it there for 20-30 seconds.

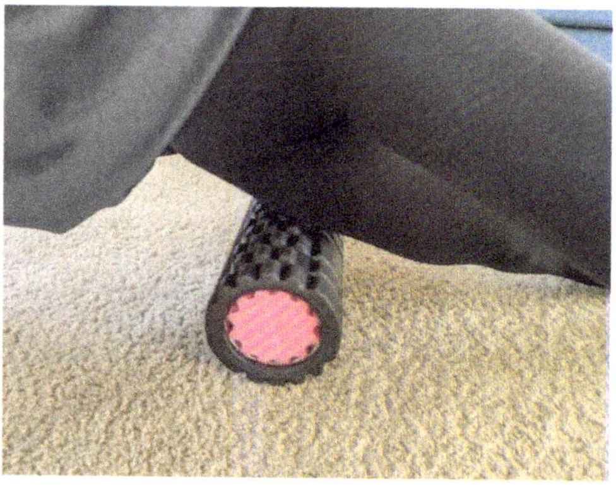

    - A hand held massage tool - these tools can help apply additional pressure to a knotted area - more than a hand can do. My favorite is a massage gun.

Athletes always want to know what they can do to keep the bones in place, permanently, so they never have such a problem again. While it would be wonderful if there were a way to ensure that the bones of the hips and low back stay in ideal approximation, the very nature of movement makes it impossible. Athletes are going to keep doing the same repetitive movements and exposing their bodies to a myriad of stressors that they can't have total control over, so hip alignment shifts from moment to moment.

The best thing an athlete can do is:

- Follow a hip stabilization exercise program on a regular basis
- Get hips aligned on a regular basis to keep alignment problems from getting out of hand and causing a serious problem
- ***If you are not getting aligned regularly - at least go when a muscle starts to feel tight

A note for people who are not competitive athletes, but have low back/groin/buttock/hip pain:

It is highly likely that your hips are out of alignment too! Outside of competitive athletics, there are lots of situations that can create a pelvic alignment problem. It can happen when you bend over and then twist when standing back up. It can happen while you're putting groceries in the car or when you step off a curb at an awkward angle. It can happen when you're just carrying kids. Everyday movement stressors can easily shift the position of these bones. So, the above recommendations for athletes apply to you as well. Getting your alignment worked on with a physical therapist or certified athletic trainer, and then following a regular hip stabilization exercise program will do wonders for keeping this problem in check.

DEEP BRUISES

Deep bruises (also called contusions) are common in the thigh, arm or calf. Contusions can come from getting kicked or from hitting someone's bent knee. In sports that involve a small but forcefully driven ball, they can occur anywhere. This is often referred to as a "dead leg" or "dead arm." A contusion is a situation where many blood vessels break, causing diffuse, long, and slow bleeding. Athletes often keep playing after the incident, but by the next morning find that they can hardly move, due to pain and stiffness. The blood pools and seeps downward, due to gravity. Sometimes discoloration is evident, but sometimes the bleeding is so deep down, you can't see discoloration on the surface. You may see swelling and skin tightness from the build up of pressure, depending on how bad it is.

Rest, ice, compression, and elevation are super important with this injury. Done quickly, they combine to great effect to minimize the extent of the bleeding, and therefore the amount of pain and swelling. Left unchecked, the bleeding can take weeks to be cleared out of the body, and often it doesn't move out. It can just pool in the area, thickening with time, which makes it more difficult for the body to cycle out.

What to do:

After any hit, even if it doesn't seem that significant:

- Ice the area for 20 minutes on, 1.5 hours off as much as possible for the next 24-72 hours.
- Use an ace bandage for compression. Wrap the bandage from below the affected area, and move toward the heart. Keep it tighter until past the

injured area, then whatever is left of the bandage can be loose. A thigh sleeve can also be used for compression. The purpose of compression is to limit the amount of blood that seeps downward, out of the original damaged area.

- Elevate - Keep it up as much as possible, in order to also limit the amount of blood that can seep downward, due to gravity.

After 24-72 hours when the bleeding is controlled:

You have to get the swelling moving out of the area, so it doesn't thicken up and just sit there! This is super important. It's also super painful, but it has to be done! You need to massage or use a roller on the affected area, moving from a point further from the heart to a point closer to the heart. Do this for a few minutes, then ice and put the sleeve or ace bandage back on. This will limit any of what you just moved out of the area to seep back down. While it is important to do this, it is also important to not get too aggressive, especially before the bleeding has been controlled, or you could end up with the development of a further problem—Myositis Ossificans.

Myositis Ossificans:

Myositis Ossificans is where bone tissue calcifies within the muscle. Sometimes with a deep bruise, the bone is bruised as well as the muscle, so there is active healing going on in both structures. In this process, some newly laid down uneven bone tissue can project into the muscle, and act as a grater as the muscle moves over the top of it. This mostly occurs in the large muscles of the arms or legs, with the quadriceps muscle on the front of the thigh being the most common location.

You can create a risk for myositis ossificans if you do not allow enough rest time following a contusion and by not taking the RICE initial treatment steps that I outlined previously. Treatment that is too aggressive also creates risk.

Symptoms of Myositis Ossificans:

- Pain and swelling that come back a few weeks after the initial injury
- Lack of improvement over a few weeks time.
- Limited range of motion.

What to do:

Treat the injury as if it were new.

- Rest
- Ice
- Compression
- Elevation
- See a sports medicine physician as soon as possible.

COMMON KNEE INJURIES

In this section, I'll describe the things you'll need to assess in a knee injury situation and then describe the kinds of injuries that can happen. With that context in mind, I'll then describe essential treatment options.

The things that need to be assessed with any knee injury are:

- Swelling
- Available range of motion (How far can they bend it and can they straighten it all the way - compared to the uninjured leg)
- Instability
- Pain

Swelling:

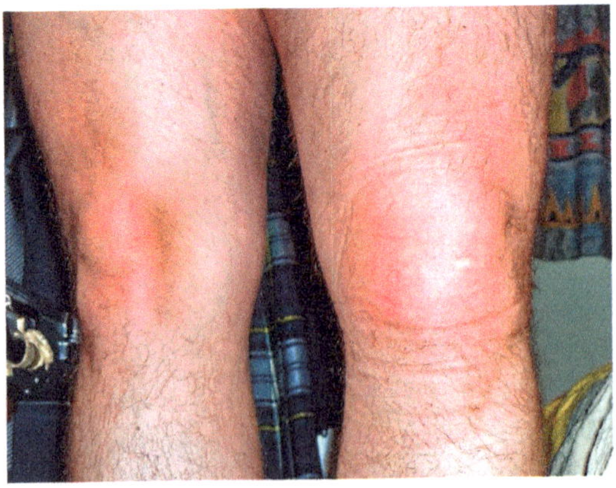

If there is a large amount of swelling that fills the whole knee, it can only be due to one of three things:
- An Anterior Cruciate Ligament (ACL) tear
- A tear of the meniscus cartilage in the outer third (where the blood supply is greater)
- A dislocated kneecap

Damage to other structures usually causes swelling in a more limited area.

Range of motion:

The restriction in range of motion is proportional to the amount of structural damage. The more restriction there is in range of motion, the more structural damage has occurred.

Instability:

Instability is the feeling of the knee buckling underneath you at unpredictable moments. It is particularly common when ligaments have been damaged, but can also occur with meniscus injuries. A picture is provided in the next section showing where the meniscus and ligaments are in the knee.

Another way instability can manifest is the necessity of walking with the leg in a certain position in order to avoid pain and buckling. The feeling of instability is disconcerting. It causes one to move slowly and desire to hold on to furniture or something that provides the stability the leg cannot. The amount of instability is also proportional to the amount of structural damage.

Pain:

Pain can be very specific to a small area or diffuse. Make a note of which seems to be the case. This will help you identify the kind of injury you're dealing with and what to do about it.

Ligament tears

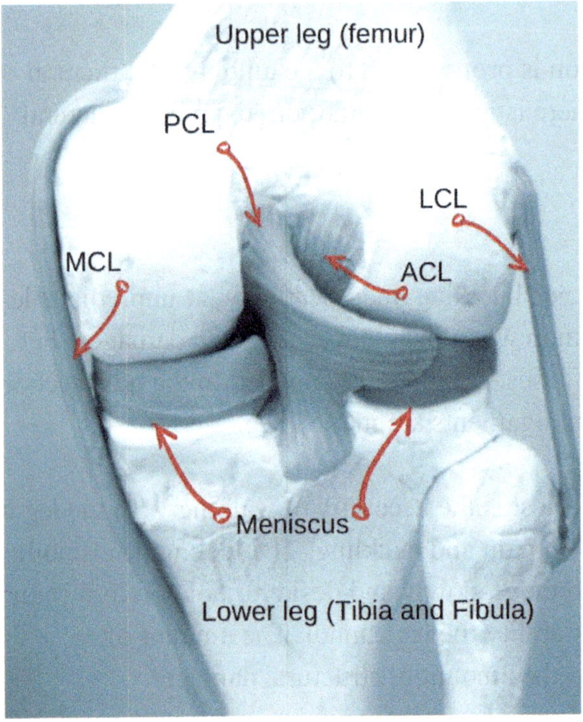

The knee from the back

Ligaments hold the bones together. The knee has 4 main ligaments—the MCL, the ACL, the PCL, and the LCL. I'll describe each of these below.

(ID 90528012 © Edward Olive| Dreamstime.com)

MCL - The MCL is located on the inside portion of the knee, the side that faces the other knee. This is commonly torn when an athlete sustains a hit on the outside of the knee while the foot is planted. An MCL tear often occurs together with a meniscus tear, as it is attached to the meniscus, and a tear of the ACL as well. This is referred to as an unhappy triad. More information about the Meniscus is provided in the next section.

If just the MCL is stretched or has small tears, swelling will be limited to the area around the damaged ligament. Pain will be specific to the site, range of motion will be somewhat limited, and there will be little instability.

The bigger an MCL tear is, the more pain, loss of motion, and instability an athlete will experience. You can recognize an MCL that is completely torn when the athlete reports a feeling of the bones swaying, unless they walk with their foot turned out.

The MCL sits outside the knee capsule, and therefore has a better blood supply than other ligaments. It is able to heal itself, given time.

ACL - The ACL crosses through the knee from front to back to stabilize the knee during cutting and twisting motions.

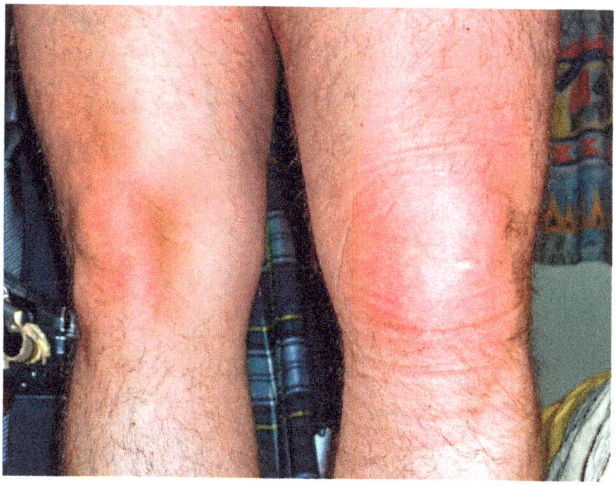

A torn ACL produces a large amount of swelling in the first several hours after injury. This can be limited through proper care, but can't be controlled altogether. If you don't make any effort to ice, compress, and elevate right after the injury, it will usually swell to an extremely uncomfortable size, due to fluid build up. This fluid has to go down, before any imaging or surgery can be done.

When the ACL is torn, swelling will build, and the available range of motion will decrease. Instability will be transient, with the knee giving out at odd moments. The athlete will report that pain seems to be everywhere.

As this ligament is inside the knee joint, the blood supply to it is not that great, and it generally is not able to heal itself. It requires surgical reconstruction.

The ACL is essential for any sport involving a lot of change of direction. If a person does not engage in such activities, it is possible to function without an intact ACL. The body will accommodate the instability over time by creating new muscle firing patterns sufficient to stabilize the knee during regular activities such as walking and running. The lack of an ACL will cause the joint surfaces to interact in a way they normally wouldn't however, which will produce a wearing down of articular cartilage (arthritis) sooner than it normally would occur.

PCL - The PCL crosses through the knee from back to front and also serves to stabilize the knee during cutting and twisting motions.

The PCL is less often injured than the ACL, as a hit or fall from the direction of force required to damage it is not as common. Due to lack of blood supply, it also generally will not heal itself. Surgery to repair this ligament is often not effective at reducing the instability, so athletes often bypass the surgery and opt to work to strengthen muscles and develop neuromuscular workarounds to produce stability as they return to play. As with the lack of an ACL, however, this will produce degeneration within the joint sooner than normal.

When the PCL is torn, swelling is general, but there tends not to be near as much as with an ACL tear. Pain, loss of range of motion and instability are also generally less than with an ACL tear.

LCL - The LCL is located on the outside portion of the knee, the side that faces away from the other knee. LCL tears are uncommon because they require a strong hit to the inside of the knee. That mechanism is simply not very common.

When the LCL is torn, swelling will be over the damaged area, and pain will be in a specific place. Instability will depend on the extent of damage.

The LCL is outside of the joint capsule, and therefore has a good blood supply. It will heal itself.

Meniscus tears

There are two menisci in the knee. They are cartilage pads that act as shock absorbers and deepen the articulating surface of the joint. Pain associated with a meniscus tear depends on how big it is, where it is, and the type of tear it is. Pain is caused by the bone picking up an edge of the tear and pinching the meniscus between the bones. After the initial inflammation from a tear calms down, it may lay down nicely on its own for a while and not cause any problem, but then act up again unexpectedly at some point in the future when the torn area again gets pinched between the bones. With any meniscus tear, there is a chance that it will tear more. It is hard to predict how much trouble a meniscus tear will cause over time.

The blood supply to the outer part of the meniscus is quite good, but for the part of the meniscus that's farther into the middle of the knee, the blood supply is actually quite poor. Surgery is a good option for some meniscus tears if they are in a place that allows the torn sides to be sewn together and get enough blood supply to heal well. Other tears will be too big or located in a part of the meniscus that won't heal well. Tears that can't be fixed are usually trimmed off, so there is not a rough edge that can be pinched between the bones.

Meniscus tears will cause pain in the joint line, the space between the upper and lower leg bones. It can also cause a clicking or catching sensation. Sometimes, the meniscus will be caught in the joint, causing it to lock up, or the knee to be unable to straighten out all the way, and cause serious pain at any effort to do it. It will usually unlock after a time of letting the surrounding musculature relax.

Combination tears:

It is quite common for an injury to involve multiple ligaments and meniscus.

What to do in the case of any knee injury:

- Ice - 20 min on, 1.5 hours off for the first 24-48 hours, top and bottom of knee preferably

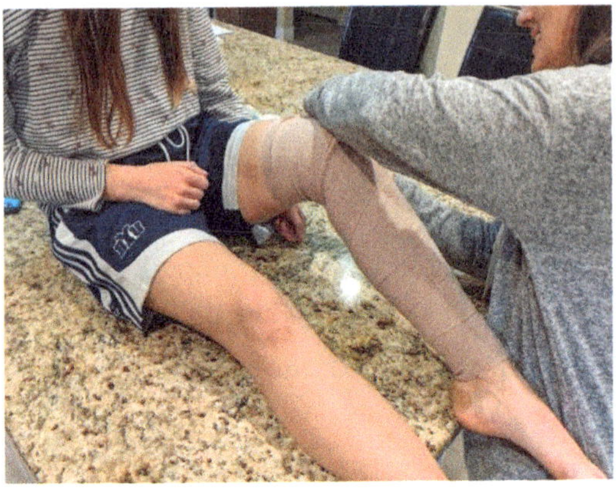

- Wrap the leg with an ace bandage. Have the athlete sit with the knee in the most comfortable position, usually a little bit bent. Start at the ankle and work your way up. Overlap each time you go around with half of the bandage. Pull the wrap to create compression from the ankle until you pass the knee joint. Whatever is left over of the bandage can just be loose. Check that the bandage is not too tight, by pinching the nail of the big toe. It will go white when you pinch it, then should return to a normal color when you let go. If it doesn't return to a normal color, or returns to color very slowly, the bandage is too tight.
  To watch a video showing how to apply an ace bandage for compression and support of a knee injury, click this link.
  https://youtu.be/oMsAURiOjj4
- Use acetaminophen for pain, not ibuprofen.
- See a sports medicine physician.

Often, a doctor will order an MRI to get a good view of the damage. In order to see most clearly inside the knee, it is best for the swelling to be minimal. All of the efforts to ice, compress, elevate and rest will pay off in being able to do the MRI, and any necessary surgery more quickly.

Patellar Tendinitis

This occurs below the kneecap, where the thigh muscles attach to the lower leg. With overuse, the muscle gets tight and pulls harder on its attachment to the bone, causing the attachment to get inflamed. It comes on gradually, being a little sore one day, and getting worse with continued activity.

What to do when this first occurs:

- Ice at the pain site for 20 minutes on, 1.5 hours off as much as possible over the next 24-48 hours.
- Massage or roll out the quads, as tight muscles are pulling on the attachment and need to be loosened up. You will likely find painful spots/bumps within the muscle. Concentrate on going over those areas. Even though this is painful, it will help a lot.

For any activity soon after the injury occurs:

- Warm up really well and stretch the quads.
- You may need to modify the amount of jumping activity, as this will aggravate it the most.
- Stay well hydrated.
- Ice after the activity for 20 minutes.

If the pain becomes chronic:

- Warm up really well and stretch the quads before any activity.
- Wear a patellar strap around the point where the tendon attaches to the lower leg bone. This limits the pulling of the tendon on the bone. Another option is to use pre-wrap, wrapped around the leg and rolled up to sit at the pain point.

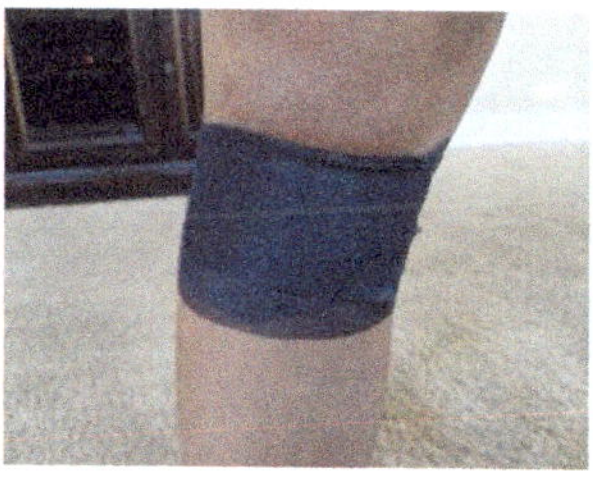
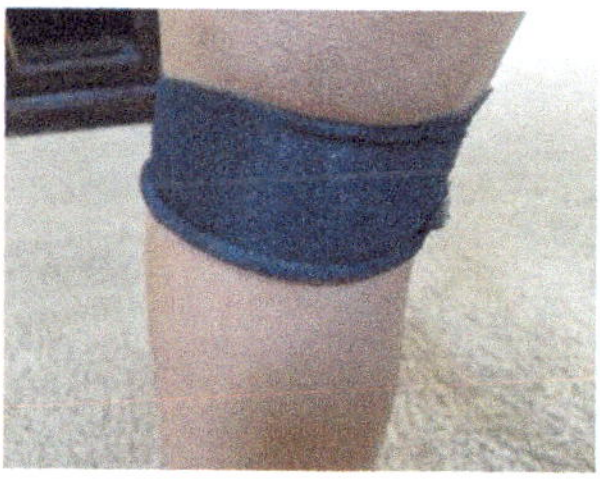
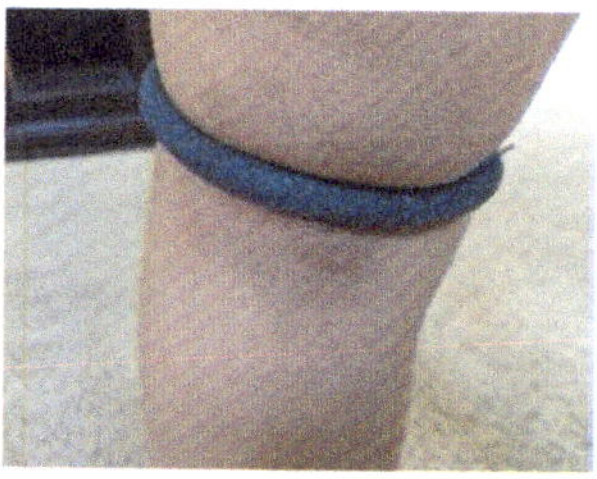

- Modify the amount of jumping activity or running.
- Ice for 20 minutes after any activity.
- See a sports medicine physician to explore options.

Osgood-Schlatter Disease

When the patellar tendon pulls on the lower leg bone at its attachment point while a teenager is in an intense growing phase, the tendon pulls away from the bone in the area of the growth plate, and the bone lays down extra calcium at the site, causing a painful bump to form. The pain usually calms down as the teenager gets through this phase, though the bump stays there.

The instructions in the previous section apply in this case as well.

SHIN SPLINTS

Shin splints occur when muscles become overly stressed and begin pulling on the connection to the bone, which causes inflammation. In chronic cases, the bone lays down extra calcium in this area, so the bone feels bumpy, instead of smooth.

While all shin splints are caused by overuse, there are a few immediate triggers for the stress the muscle-to-bone connection experiences:

- A recent increase in the intensity or amount of activity.
- The structure of the foot causes force to be distributed up the leg disproportionately through the shin area. This is quite likely the trigger if the shin splints are in both legs.
- Weakness or tightness of hip and lower leg muscles may cause extra force to be distributed through the shin area

What to do:

Getting rid of shin splints once you have them is difficult, so prevention is the best option. If you are going to start up with exercise or training after an extended time off, allow yourself to gradually build up both the amount of time and the intensity of your activity. 1-2 weeks of gradual build up is a good rule of thumb. Warm up, cool down, and stretch the calves well. Also, make sure you aren't wearing worn out shoes. Shoes need good arch support.

If shin pain has just started:

- Ice for 20 minutes on and 1.5 hours off (as much as possible) for the first 24-48 hours.
- Limit activity in order to get this to calm down.
- Roll out shins and calves.
- Look for structural reasons why this could be happening:

  Look at the feet. Are the arches flat? Does the back of the foot roll inward (look from behind while the heel is flat on the floor)? If this is the case, you need a good pair of insoles. Start with regular insoles available at pharmacies or online stores. If this helps some, but not enough, you can move up to custom fit, moldable insoles or orthotics. At this point, you need to get some help from an athletic trainer, a physical therapist, or a sports medicine physician.

If shin pain is chronic - you rest it goes away, you do any activity it comes back:

Before any activity:

- Warm up
- Roll out shins and calves
- If you are in a situation where you need to compete - get through a season, a big game, etc. - then you can tape your arches and/or shins. Shins are difficult to keep taping, because the tape has to be applied directly on the skin. When you take the tape off, it pulls off skin cells, leaving the skin red, raw and sensitive.

After any activity:

- Ice for 20 minutes
- Roll out shins and calves

Chronic shin pain is always due to structural issues. Custom fit moldable insoles or orthotics can help this problem, as can a lot of work on foot and ankle biomechanics. See a sports medicine physician as soon as possible. Without intervention, this problem will not go away.

COMMON ANKLE INJURIES

The most common sports injury is an ankle sprain. Ankle sprains can happen when you jump and land on someone else's foot, or when someone slides into you when your foot is planted. They can happen when a field is uneven and you step in a hole. . . The list goes on. What essentially happens, though, is that the ankle joint is forced into a position that is past where it's normal range of motion allows it go, and the ligaments that attach the bones to each other get stretched and torn.

The outside of the ankle, also called the lateral side, is more vulnerable to sprains than the inside. This is because the movements that stretch the outside ligaments are more common, and because the structure of the outside of the ankle simply allows for more movement. More movement is important for many sport-related movements, but it means there is also less stability. The inside of the ankle is covered by one thick ligament, which is more difficult to tear, and not exposed as often to enough force to tear it. The outside has three smaller separate ligaments. The front most ligament, the talofibular or TFL, gets impacted the most, and is usually torn when the foot is pointed down and to the inside when weight gets put on it.

There are three degrees of ligament damage.
1st degree - stretched, with small tears
2nd degree - partly torn
3rd degree - completely torn

How to evaluate any ankle injury:

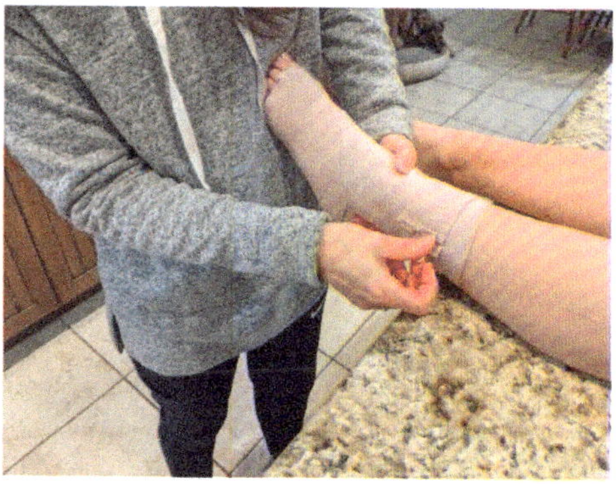

Keep in mind that an injured ankle could have a fractured bone as well as damaged ligaments.

The basic things to check for include:

- Is the athlete able to put weight on the ankle? If it's too painful to put weight on and the pain shoots up the leg, that is an indication of a fracture.
- How limited is the range of motion? If the athlete has very little motion and motion causes a lot of pain, this may also be an indication of a fracture. Keep in mind that motion might be limited in one direction, but not others.
- How much pain does the athlete report? Major pain, especially when just sitting there may indicate a fracture.
- How much swelling is present? If there is still a significant amount of swelling after resting, icing, compression, and elevation, fracture is a possibility
- Bruising - this will take a day or two to show up, but it signifies that structures have been broken/torn and blood has seeped out into the surrounding area.

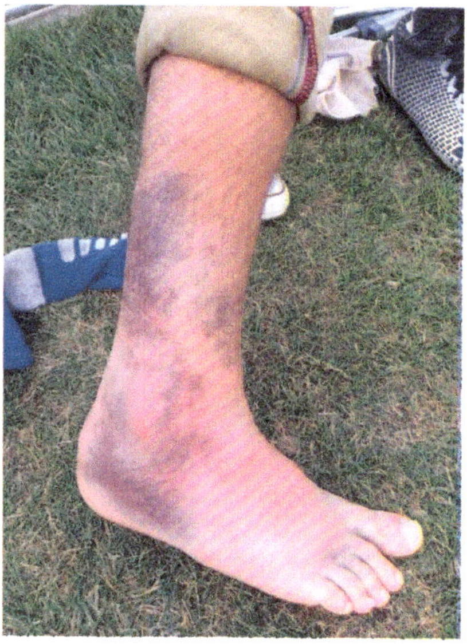

In the case of any of the above, you should see a sports medicine physician as soon as you can get an appointment to check for fracture and assess the extent of the ligament damage. The ankle will for sure need physical therapy, after the break heals, or immediately if there's no break.

What to do in the first 24-72 hours:

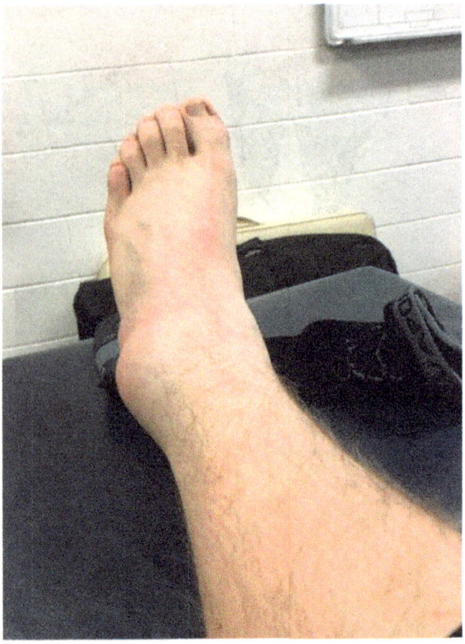

- Rest. Use crutches if putting weight on the ankle is painful enough that it affects your ability to walk normally. If your daily routine requires a lot of moving around, crutches are especially important.
- Ice - 20 min on, 1.5 hours off.
- Wrap with an ace bandage, starting at the toes. Overlap each time you go around with half of the bandage. Pull the wrap to create compression from the toes until you pass the ankle joint. Whatever is left over of the bandage can just be loose. Check that the bandage is not too tight, by pinching the nail of the big toe. It will go white when you pinch it, but it should immediately go back to it's normal color when you let go. If it doesn't, or normal color returns slowly, the bandage is too tight.
  Click the link to watch a video showing how to apply an ace wrap for compression and support of an ankle injury.
  https://youtu.be/UmcSrN99_Qw
- Use acetaminophen for pain, not ibuprofen.
- Elevate the ankle.

If the ankle doesn't swell much, the range of motion is not very limited, and pain and motion improve over the next few days, you can avoid a trip to the doctor. Even in this case, physical therapy is still a good idea for a few reasons:

Ligaments take a long time to heal. Though you may be able to do normal activity, and not notice any problems, ligaments go through a process of remodeling that lasts many months after injury. During this time, they are more vulnerable to reinjury.

Damaged ligamentous tissue is filled in with scar tissue, which is not as strong or flexible as the original tissue. Also, stretched ligaments stay stretched out. These two things predispose the ligaments to reinjury.

Finally, ligaments have structures within them that send information to your brain about where your foot is in space and in time. When ligaments are damaged, that information pathway is disrupted, leaving the ligaments prone to reinjury due to lack of coordination. Work in therapy is done to help re-establish normal communication pathways to the brain. This retraining is critical to preventing reinjury.

BLISTERS

Blisters are common and don't usually create a serious problem, but they can be intensely painful! The best thing to do is avoid them in the first place, which is entirely doable. Blisters form in very predictable situations.

Prevention:

Situations that produce blisters:

- Whenever an athlete begins wearing new cleats or new shoes of any kind
- When undertaking a new and unfamiliar activity
- The start of a new season after having time off
- Any activity that lasts for a long time

What you can do:

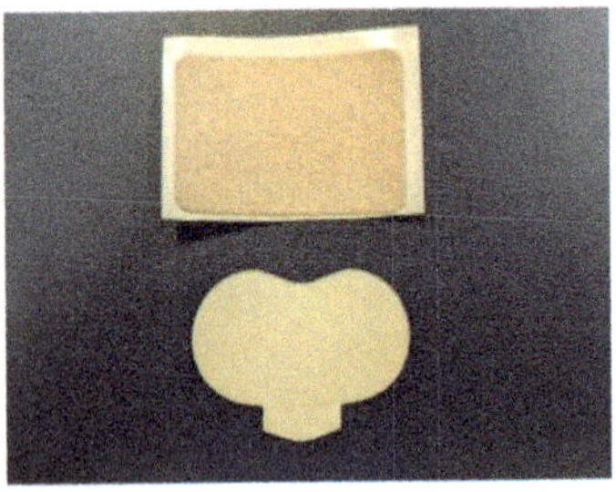

- Use Blister foam - a peel-off, stick-on, thin piece of foam made particularly in the shape of the back of the heel. They work great, but they're expensive.
- Use moleskin - a soft piece of fabric with a sticky back. Cut to fit the area, peel off and stick on the skin.
- Use New Skin - a liquid you can put over an area when you start feeling the friction which will dry and act as a protective barrier

After you've got a blister:

What to do:

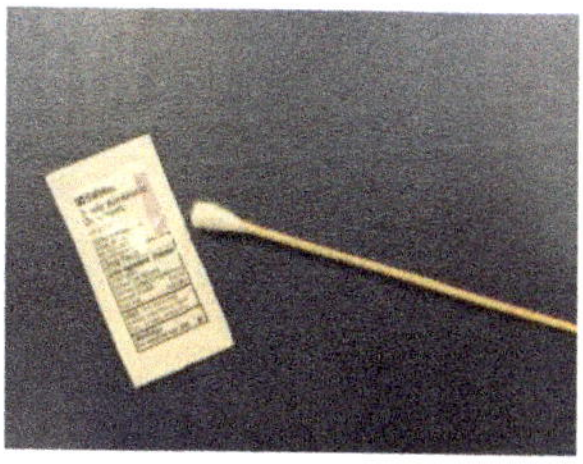

- If the blister is not aggravated by normal footwear, leave them intact and let the body drain them in a natural way.
- If the blister is in a place where it is aggravated by normal footwear, it needs to be popped. The best thing to use to pop them is a one time use lancet (to avoid infection). Twist off the cap and use the sharp end to puncture the blister. Drain with gauze or tissue. Squeeze the fluid out. Dry off.
- Clean with soap and water or an antiseptic liquid.
- Apply antibiotic ointment.
- Cover with a band-aid to keep the ointment from rubbing off.
- Re-apply ointment several times over the next day or two.

To cover for playing sports or dancing:

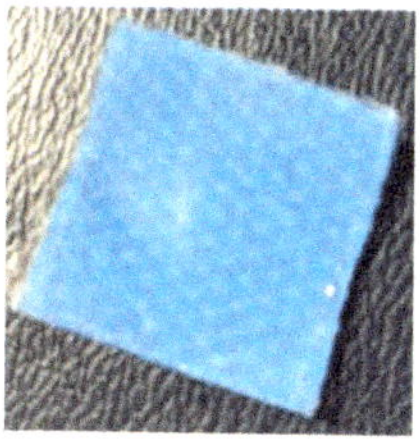

- Use a gel square to cover the blister.
- Cover the gel square with a band-aid, or piece of moleskin, depending on where it is.
- Tape over that with pre-wrap and stretchy tape. The tape should touch skin above and below, to keep everything in place.

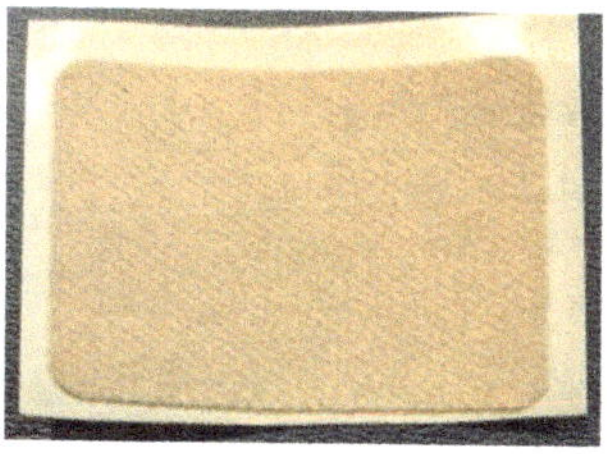

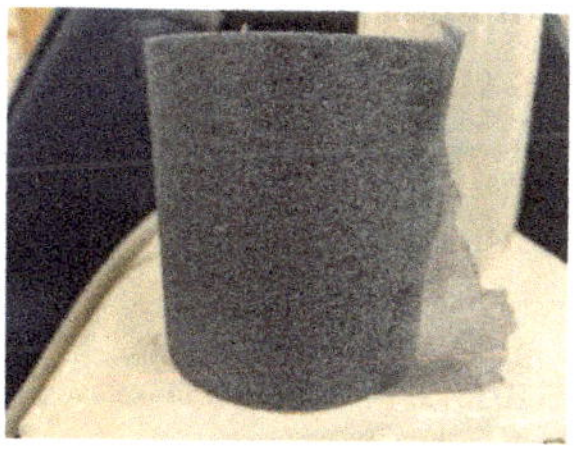

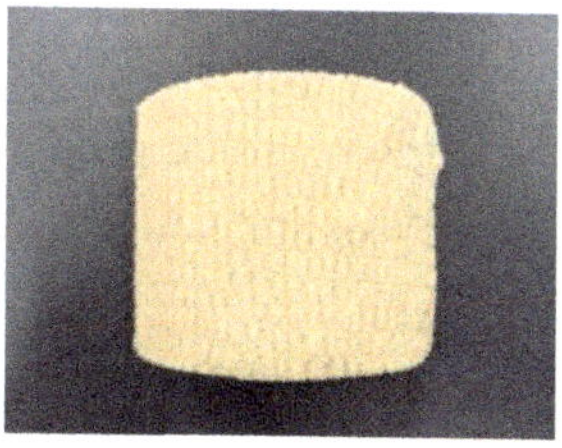

BRUISED TOENAILS

When athletes get their toes stomped on, particularly by someone wearing cleats, blood vessels under the toenail break, and blood can pool underneath the nail, causing a build up of pressure. This is also common when running long distances with a lot of downhill time, as the big toe jams up against the front of the shoe.

What to do:

- Ice several times during the first 24 hours afterward. This may keep it from bleeding so much that the associated pressure becomes unbearable.

If the pressure causes too much pain:

- Release the pressure by poking a hole in the toenail to drain out the blood.
- Use a one time use lancet. (Pictured here) Twist off the cap and heat the sharp end with a lighter. This will make it go in easily.

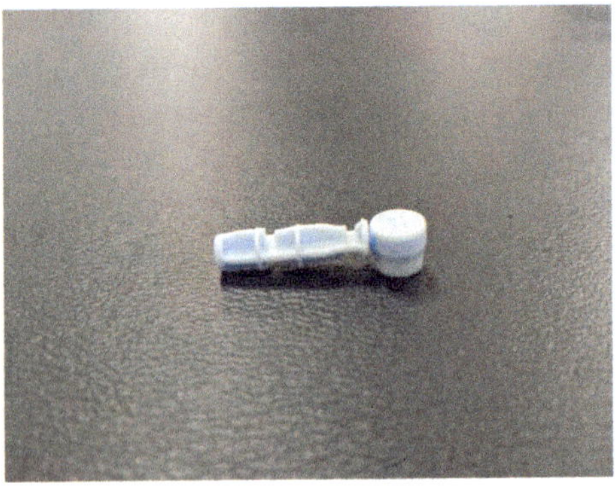

- Have some gauze or tissues ready.
- Puncture through the nail and drain the blood out. This can squirt, so be prepared.
- Push and squeeze to get out all you can.
- Cover the puncture entrance with antibacterial ointment
- Cover with a band-aid.

Toenails in this situation will often, over time, detach from the nailbed and fall off. It is best to keep the toenail on as long as possible, to help protect a new toenail growing underneath. The old toenail can be somewhat loose and snag on socks, so it helps to tape the toenail down to hold it in place until it is ready to fall off.

DEHYDRATION AND HEAT ILLNESS

Dehydration:

Dehydration occurs when you lose significantly more fluid from the body than you take in. Dehydration prevents body processes from their normal function. Dehydration is not just a lack of fluids, but also a lack of minerals known as electrolytes. Studies show that a loss of as little as 2% of body weight as sweat can cause a noticeable decrease in physical and mental performance. Losses of 5% or more can actually limit work capacity by as much as 30%. (http://sportscardiologybc.org/the-effects-of-hydration-on-athletic-performance/)

If kids understand that the result of not putting in the effort to hydrate well is definitely going to show up in their performance level, they pay a bit more attention. Frequently, when blaming their unhappiness with their performance on things such as the coach unaccountably pulling them out, or choosing someone else to execute an important play - their attention should be brought back to that decrease in physical and mental performance caused by a small amount of dehydration. Doing everything you can possibly do to perform at your best, is the hallmark of a great athlete.

The effects of dehydration can be counteracted by hydrating well ahead of activity, having a plan to replace fluid and electrolytes during activity and following through on it. It also means making serious efforts to rehydrate after activity. Having a plan includes keeping track of body weight before and after activity, so you know how much weight was lost in order to rehydrate enough after activity.

As a parent you can model this behavior for your children, and you can help them create habits that will serve them well as they get older.

To make this simple and actionable use the following guidelines for intense or extended athletic activities like games and practices:

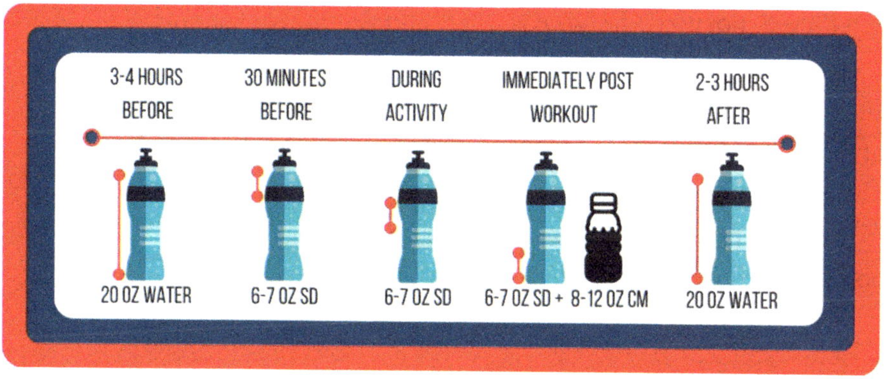

- Get a 20 ounce see-through water bottle that the athlete will always use for this purpose.
- Drink the whole thing full of water 3-4 hours before activity - with food.
- From here on through the activity and immediately post activity it should be some kind of sports drink, not water, as they need the electrolytes and the sugar. I have many athletes who don't like drinking sports drinks. If they insist on drinking water, then they need to supplement electrolytes in some other way. I have them take a little bit of the concentrated electrolyte add-in mixed with water, then wash it down with more water, and use some chews or goo to give them some sugar.
- During warm-up or 30 minutes before, drink ⅓ of the bottle.
- During activity drink ⅓ of the bottle during half time or other breaks.
- Immediately post activity, drink 8-12 oz of chocolate milk and ⅓ bottle of sports drink. (The chocolate milk is important because it contains protein as well as carbohydrate. The protein helps increase the body's uptake of carbohydrate, replenishing used energy stores.)

- In the following 2-3 hours drink the whole 20 oz water bottle at least once, with food. If they have been playing in the heat and have sweated a lot, drink another whole 20 oz.

Based on the recommendations of the American College of Sports Medicine https://www.researchgate.net/publication/6526394_American_College_of_Sports_Medicine_position_stand_Exercise_and_Fluid_Replacement

If you can remember to get the athlete to step on a scale at least a time or two before activity, and then again afterward, you will get a good idea of how much they lose on a regular basis, and use that as a more accurate measure to go by for how much to drink following activity. The amount to drink is one 20 oz bottle for every pound lost.

Heat Illness:

One problem with dehydration is that it hampers the body's ability to regulate temperature, so it is often a contributor to heat illness. While we are more aware of the possibility of problems that might arise in hot and humid environments, heat illness can also happen at lower temperatures. The key to being able to exercise in any environment is being acclimatized, a process which can take a couple of weeks. Therefore, be more aware of problems that can occur due to heat when traveling to compete away from home, especially if the climate is much different than where you live. Also, problems are more likely to occur when returning to intense activity after some time off. Tryouts after an off season are an example.

Heat Cramps:

Heat cramps usually happen in the calves or the hamstrings, due to fatigue and dehydration. The thinking is that a depletion of salt in the system leaves muscles unable to fully relax. Some people don't seem to ever get cramps, while others seem especially prone to them. One theory is that the people who are prone to cramping are "salty sweaters", meaning their sweat contains a greater concentration of salt than people who aren't prone to them.

You've likely heard of people drinking pickle juice as an anti-cramping strategy, as pickle juice contains a large amount of salt. While I can't say for absolute certain this works or it doesn't, it is rather unlikely to be a remedy of choice for many people.

The best strategy is prevention, instead of intervention. Since cramping tends to happen to certain people, they can take steps to avoid it. Also, it's a good idea to take preventative measures when the stakes are higher - important games, situations when athletes are unlikely to be able to take a break, activity in hot and humid climates are examples.

Prevention:

- Hydrate ahead of intense or extended activity (see the hydration guidelines above).
- Take slow release electrolyte tablets before intense or extended activity. I give my athletes a product called Heat Guard.
- Drink a sports drink during breaks and after activity to help rehydrate.
- Eat a snack size Payday or Salted Nut Roll during a mid activity break. This will provide salt, sugar, and protein.

When cramps come on:

- Stop activity
- Use a highly concentrated electrolyte replenishment solution mixed with water - my strategy is to have the athlete drink the concentrated solution with a small amount of water. This tastes awful, but they can down it quickly. Then the athlete can drink more regular water or a

sports drink to wash it down. I use a concentrated solution called Elite Electrolyte Add-In. It only takes a few drops to provide the needed replenishment.

- Stretch the problematic muscle.
- Roll out or massage the area.
- If the activity is still ongoing, after the athlete has had 15 or 20 minutes to get some of the solution into their system, and the athlete feels well enough to return, then they can go ahead and try.

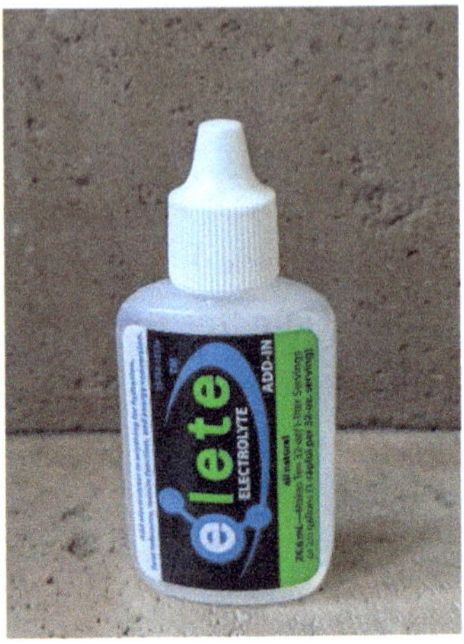

Heat Exhaustion:

Heat exhaustion is quite common in sports activity, but also can happen doing things like playing at the park in the summer, or standing in line at an amusement park, being in the sun for long periods of time, or hiking. Heat exhaustion usually happens when someone is active and becomes dehydrated in weather conditions that make it hard for the body to cool off. If exposure to heat is not stopped, the condition can progress to heat stroke.

Signs and Symptoms of Heat Exhaustion:

- Heavy sweating
- Cold, pale, clammy skin
- Fast, weak pulse
- Nausea or vomiting
- Muscle cramps
- Tiredness or weakness
- Dizziness
- Headache
- Fainting

Headache and a general sense of not feeling good are usually the first symptoms to show up.

What to do:

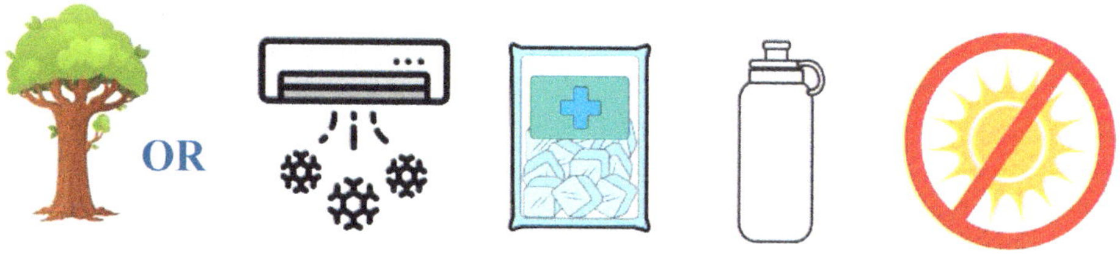

- Get out of the heat (get in the shade at the very least, but somewhere air conditioned is better). The person needs to cool down quickly.
- Put ice on the sides of the head and under the armpits. Those are strategic places that will cool the blood down more quickly.
- Drink water or a sports drink. If drinking water, eat a snack as well to get electrolytes and nutrients.
- Avoid sun exposure and physical activity for the rest of the day. It takes a while to stabilize body temperature regulation and recover energy.
- If symptoms persist longer than one hour or get worse, go to the ER.

Heat Stroke:

Heat stroke is an absolute emergency situation. The body has lost its ability to regulate temperature, causing the body's natural cooling mechanisms to fail. When body temperature gets too high, damage to body organs can occur. This can be fatal.

Signs and symptoms:

- Body temperature of 103 or higher (To be accurate, this measurement needs to be taken with a rectal thermometer. Obviously, this is not something you will be able to assess in the moment.)
- Hot, dry, red skin
- Fast, strong pulse
- Headache
- Dizziness
- Nausea
- Confusion
- Fainting

You notice that some of these symptoms are the same as those for heat exhaustion - generally, they are on a continuum, so the person will progress from heat exhaustion to heat stroke if intervention does not happen to bring the body temperature down. **One primary indicator that a person is progressing into heat stroke will be the feel of the skin. It will be hot and dry vs cold and clammy. A marked deterioration in the level of mental function is also a warning sign.**

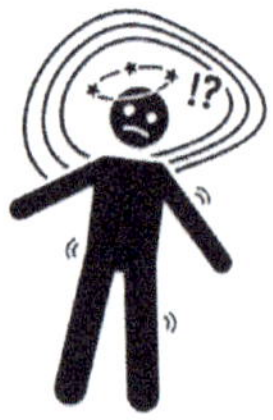

What to do:

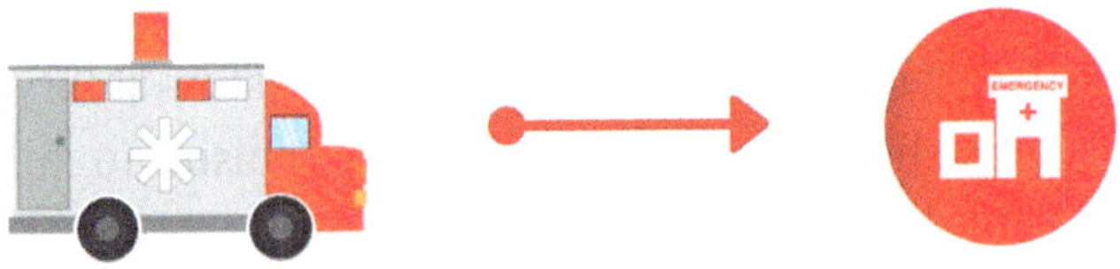

- If the athlete is at all confused or dizzy and the skin is hot and dry, call an ambulance!

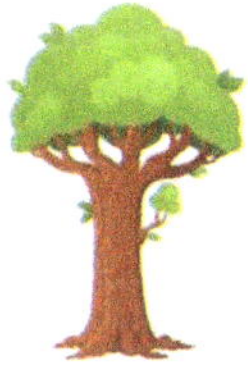

OR

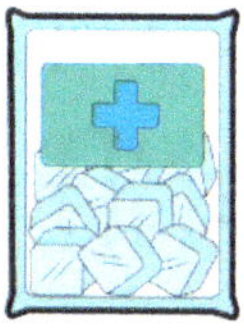

- Get out of the heat
- Pack ice or cold packs on the sides of their head, under the armpits and on their chest.
- Don’t try to get them to drink or eat anything

CUTS, LACERATIONS, AND ABRASIONS

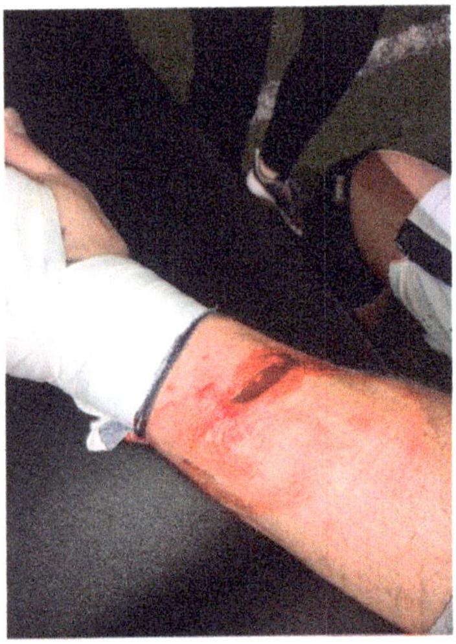

Cut: A narrow incision in the skin made by something sharp. The edges are straight.

Laceration: A wound that is produced by the tearing of soft body tissue. This type of wound is
often irregular and jagged.

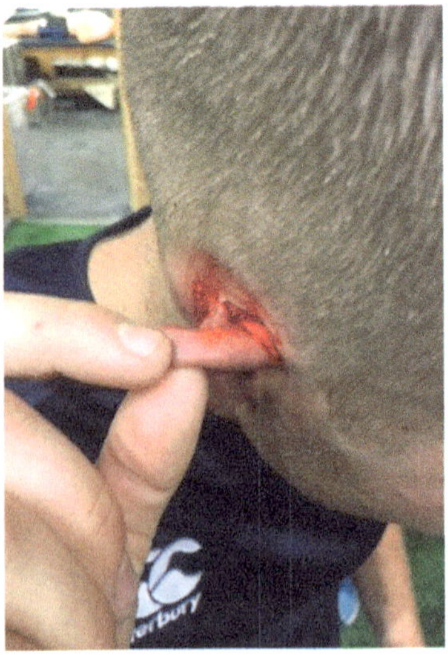

What to do:

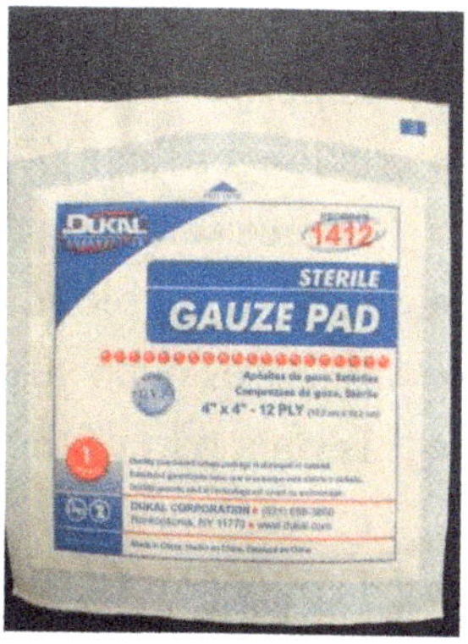

- Stop the bleeding by placing direct pressure over the wound. Using gauze is the best and the cleanest way to do this. Keep a first aid kit with you for such purposes.
- Elevate the body part above the heart to aid in stopping the bleeding.
- Keep applying new pieces of gauze on top of each other if blood soaks through. **Don't remove one piece to use another.**
- When the bleeding has stopped, clean the wound with something antibacterial or soap and water. This will always hurt - there isn't much you can do about that. But it is absolutely essential that you do a thorough job of it, especially if the injury occured on indoor artificial turf! That stuff gets nasty, and can cause serious infections.

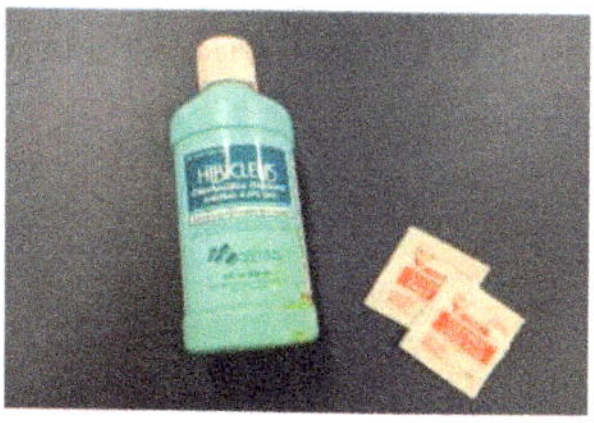

- Decide if the wound needs stitches

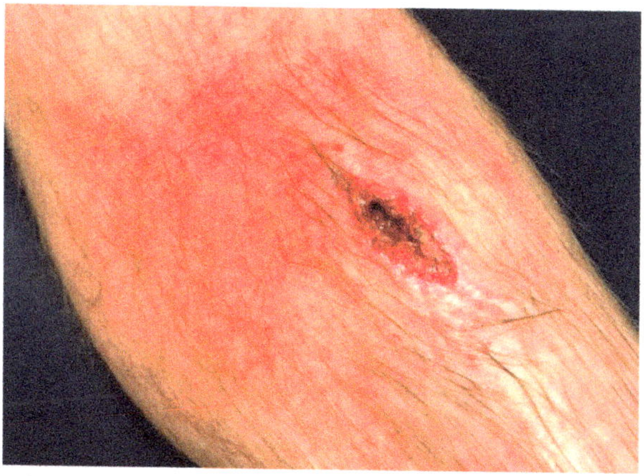

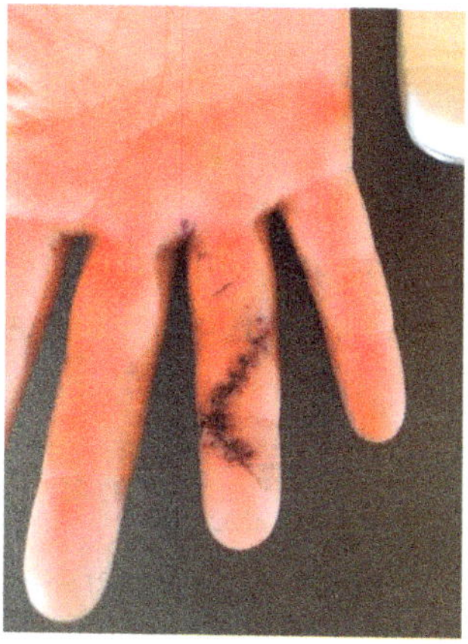

A wound needs stitches when it:

- Is deeper than ¼”
- Is longer than ½”
- Bleeds without stopping after 10 min of direct pressure
- Is spurting blood
- Exposes deep structures like bones, muscles, or tendons
- Is on a part of the body that moves - edges get pulled apart by movement
- Is on a part of the body that is hard to pull the edges together and have them stay, due to body contours, hair, or jagged edges that makes approximation difficult to hold together
- Is on the face. Stitches can help to minimize scarring.

** If stitches are needed, get them within 6-8 hours after injury.

In the meantime:

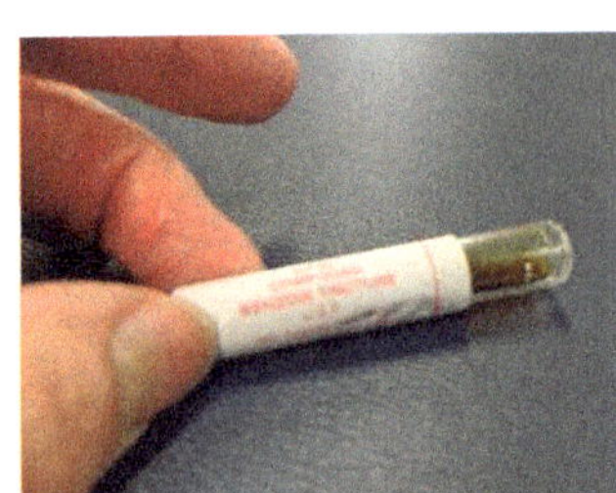

- Swab Benzoin Tincture around the wound. This is an antiseptic and will also make the area sticky, so bandages will stick better. Benzoin Tincture is usually delivered in a small plastic pod. The pod holds the chemical and when you break it, it soaks a built in piece of cotton.
- Pull the edges of the wound together as best you can using butterfly bandages or steri-strips.
- Cover the wound with stretchy coban (a kind of tape that only sticks to itself.)
- Go to the Instacare or ER, or a doctor if you can get in quickly enough.

If stitches aren't needed:

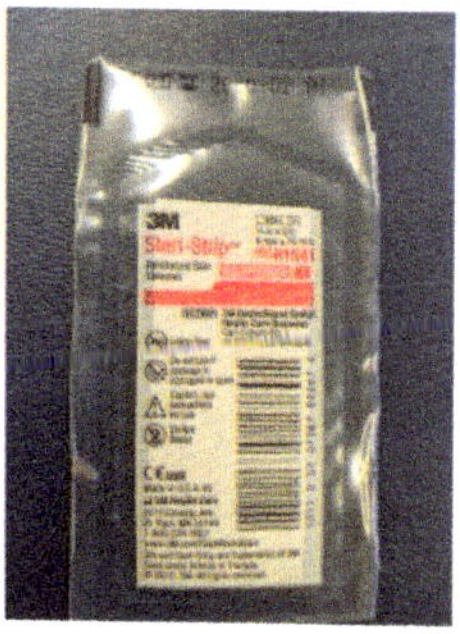

- Swab the wound with Benzoin Tincture. See the note above on how to apply.
- Pull the edges of the wound together as best you can using butterfly bandages or steri-strips.
- Cover the wound with stretchy coban. (a kind of tape that only sticks to itself)
- Don't take the steri-strips off. Just let them fall off over time.

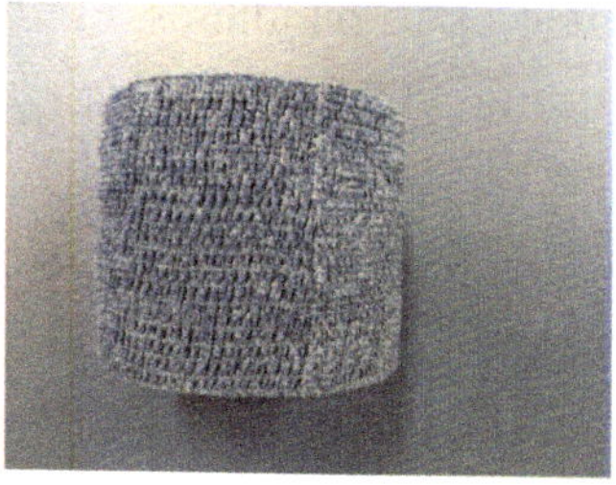

For a small superficial cut:

- Put antibiotic ointment on the wound.
- Use super glue (yes, just normal glue) to hold it together.

Abrasion: A wearing, grinding, or rubbing away by friction.

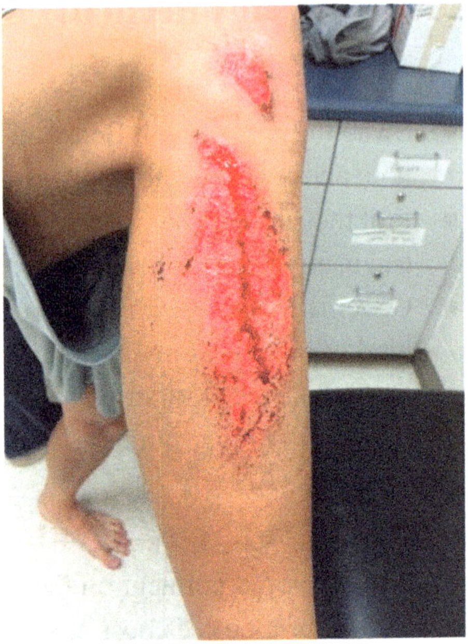

Abrasions weep - fluid seeps out of damaged blood vessels for several hours after an injury. This will stick to bandages, clothes, bedding, etc. and will be ripped off with the removal of what they are attached to. This starts the process all over again.

What to do:

- Clean the abrasion with an antibacterial cleaner, or soap and water. Do a good job of cleaning, especially if the wound happened on indoor artificial turf!
- Put antibiotic ointment on it.
- Cover with a non-stick (Telfa) pad to keep the wound from sticking to clothes. Even with a non-stick pad, it may still stick, depending on how much has seeped out. I advise removing the pad in the shower.
- Cover with stretchy coban (a kind of tape that only sticks to itself)
- When possible, allow the wound to be in the air and dry out, but put antibacterial ointment on it and cover it at night.

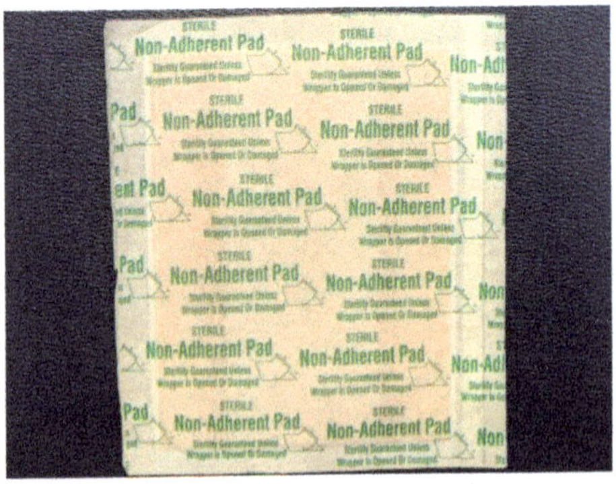

In order to play while an abrasion is still healing:

It is important to cover abrasions while playing, so they don't just reopen. This is especially important if the athlete is playing on artificial turf. Cover abrasions with non-stick pads and stretchy coban. Wear socks, long pants or a long sleeve shirt to help cover the area.

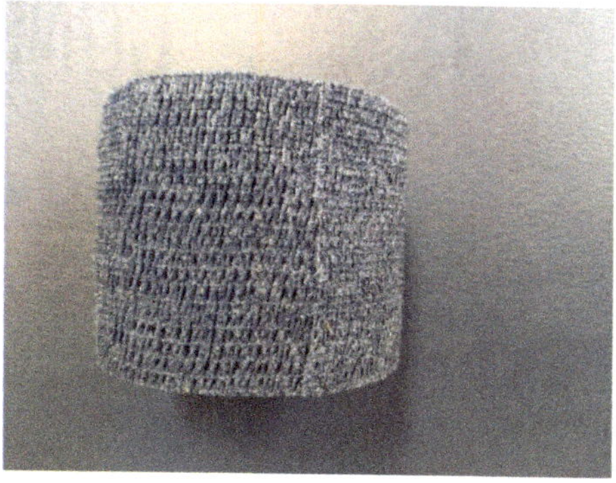

CONCLUSION

There you have it, the basics of Sports Medicine, boiled down to practical steps you can follow at home to take care of any injury, and set up the best set of circumstances you can for proceeding with healing.

By following these steps, you will provide the best care for your young athletes at home, and know when to seek out professional medical care based on the true need for it. Though any time your child sustains an injury will be stressful, you won't be left making decisions based on the lack of knowledge of what to do and the fear of not doing enough. Your confidence will reassure your child, lessening the fear and anxiety for them too.

While you never know what circumstances you will encounter with your kids, you will always have this information as a resource in the moment it's needed and to refer back to as you deal with whatever crazy situations arise. Kids are an adventure, and injuries provide some valuable lessons for them and for you. Use this information to help your child avoid what injuries you can, and then feel confident that you can take care of whatever happens that's unavoidable.

Wishing you the best of luck!